Northeast
Waterways

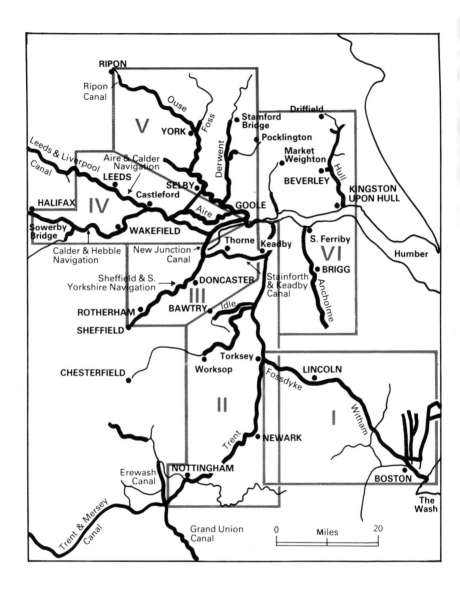

I. The Witham and Fossdyke
II. The River Trent
III. The Sheffield and South Yorkshire Navigation
IV. The Aire and Calder Navigation
V. The Yorkshire Ouse
VI. The Rivers Ancholme and the Hull via the River Humber

Northeast Waterways

*A cruising guide to
the Rivers Witham, Trent, Yorkshire
Ouse and associated waterways*

DEREK BOWSKILL

Imray Laurie Norie & Wilson Ltd
St Ives Huntingdon Cambridgeshire England

Published by
Imray, Laurie, Norie & Wilson Ltd
Wych House, St. Ives, Huntingdon,
Cambridgeshire PE17 4BT, England.

British Library Cataloguing in Publication Data

Bowskill, Derek
    Northeast waterways.
    1. Inland navigation — England, Northern
    I. Title
    386'.09428   HE436.Z4N6
    ISBN 0-85288-099-5

CAUTION
Whilst every care has been taken to ensure accuracy, neither the Publishers nor the Author will hold themselves responsible for errors, omissions or alterations in this publication. They will at all times be grateful to receive information which tends to the improvement of the work.

Printed at The Bath Press, Avon

FOREWORD

I wintered on board *Valcon* in Sheffield Canal Basin about a decade ago. *Valcon* was iced in, until after the morning ritual with a heavy-duty boathook; the basin was iced up and once I fell through the ice and bruised more ribs than ever existed in *Gray's Anatomy;* and the canal system itself fell about and was so thoroughly overcome by ice and snow, floods, Acts of God, lockouts and a general water board strike that it was not until July that I made it across the last pound at the bottom of the Tinsley Flight and then only on the third attempt at some near-flash flooding.

However, that experience did little to discourage me from enjoying the navigation when I returned to it some five years later; and that little was no more than a sensible reminder not to tie up anywhere in the centre of Rotherham. Nor was I put off the rivers by my vividly remembered experiences of the eagre (eager, aegre, aegir or bore) on the banks of the River Trent by the then novel and bravely experimental bascule bridge of King George at Keadby.

It was therefore with nothing but good feelings that I approached the research for this volume; a project covering that vast network of natural, aided and also completely artificial becks, streams, rivers and canals that go to make up the northeast waterways: from Boston to Lincoln, Torksey and Nottingham; from Stockwith to Bawtry and Worksop; from Keadby and Goole to Doncaster, Sheffield, Castleford, Leeds, Wakefield and Sowerby Bridge; from Driffield Navigation to Kingston-upon-Hull and from Brandy Wharf to South Ferriby; and with a passing glance at the Market Weighton Canal, from Trent Falls to Selby, York and Ripon – and from Barmby to Sutton and Pocklington. Over the hundreds of miles that can be cruised, there are delights and contrasts to be found in such profusion that they defy ever being comprehensively named or numbered.

What is more, these delights and contrasts are not vested only in views, places, events and things; they are also to be found in equal profusion in those men and women whose work, interest and pleasure, overwhelming passion or merely idle curiosity takes them on or close to the waterways. So many of them helped me over days, weeks and months; over miles and knots, and locks and bridges; over ups and downs, and ins and outs; over shoals and deeps, and bights and nesses; and over all the ebbing and flowing, afloat and ashore, that takes place in and around the proliferating pubs, clubs and wheelhouses . . and often down below.

To single out a few for special mention would be, by implication, to diminish the rest; and that I have no intention of doing; my thanks to you all.

Derek Bowskill
Pool in Wharfedale January 1986

ACKNOWLEDGEMENTS

I would like to offer thanks of an entirely different kind to Alex McMullen of *Motor Boat & Yachting* and Chris Bye of *The Yorkshire Post*. Thanks to their personal interest and professional commissions I was encouraged to 'keep at it' during some exceptionally long winter spells when living on board *Valcon* on a frozen-over canal did seem at times to smack more of madness and masochism than of sense or sensibility.

Without that encouragement, it is possible that I should not have stayed the course and would not have emerged knowing that the drawbacks are as nought when compared with the essence of the true experience, which is one of magic and mystery.

This guide has been produced with the co-operation of the British Waterways Board. The publishers and the author would like to thank all those members of the Board's staff who have, over the years, offered themselves well beyond the calls of duty or the demands of office. Thanks to their efforts, both *Valcon* and this volume have had their passages eased and speeded along their ways.

CONTENTS

Forward
Acknowledgements

Introduction, 3
    Table of distances – Main routes, 4
    Authorities, 5
    Key to symbols, 7
    Tidal differences, 8
    British Waterways Board Code of Conduct, 9
    Sanitary stations, 14
    BWB Water points, 14
    VHF radio, 15
    Pleasure boat licences, 16
    Recommended reading, 16
    Wharves in use for freight, 1
    Conversion tables, 21

I.   The Witham and the Fossdyke, 23
       The Witham Navigable Drains, 58

II.   The River Trent, 61
       The River Idle, 97
       The Chesterfield Canal, 101

III.   The Sheffield & South Yorkshire Navigation, 103
       The Stainforth & Keadby Canal, 103
       The New Junction, 118
       The Sheffield & South Yorkshire, 122

IV.   The Aire & Calder Navigation, 141
       The Calder & Hebble Navigation, 164
       The Selby Canal, 174

V.   The Yorkshire Ouse, 177
       The Tidal Ouse, 177
       The River Derwent and the Pocklington Canal, 213

VI.   The Rivers Ancholme and Hull via the River Humber, 219

Index, 247

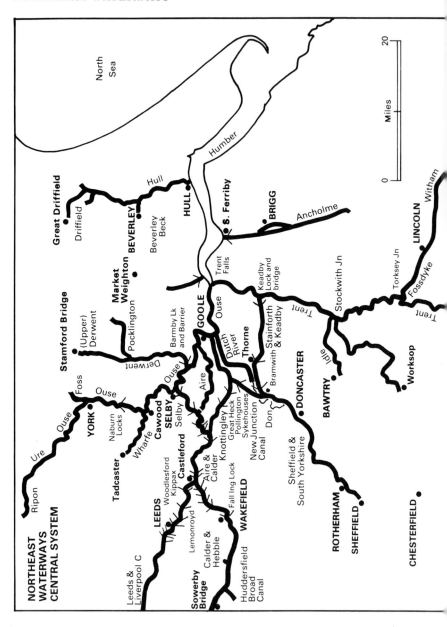

INTRODUCTION

It is hoped that this cruising guide will be of use and interest to all those who are attracted by the waterways of the northeast, whether to provide a relaxing, fireside read in the wintertime; a persuasive springtime planning aid for the next summer's season; or a handy wheelhouse book of reference for consultation while out and about on the job.

Two kinds of information are offered: hard facts and soft comment. The sketch maps, chartlets and collated facts and figures about bridges, locks and actual places are all intended to be no more and no less than accurately factual; while much of the general text and many of the illustrations are meant to offer something of the spirit and flavour of the area, location or waterway, and, as such, are subjective assessments, presented as a result of the author's personal experience.

That personal experience was gained, in the main, while piloting the author's motor-sailer around the system over the past four years. *Valcon* was built on the lines of a traditional, Scottish MFV, and when she was commissioned in 1964 it was for a life on the North Sea, and not at all for inland waterways. However, with her masts down, sails stowed, everything heavily guarded and filtered, and dressed over-all, not with flags or bunting, but with sturdy fenders, she made a resolute attack hither and yon; and while some sections of the Witham and Fossdyke and Sheffield & South Yorkshire Navigations regularly brought the tedious embarrassment of close encounters with the bottom, the draught that caused them was by no means an *embarras de richesse* when working the Yorkshire Ouse, the Trent or the Humber.

Valcon, with her 35' length x 12'6" beam x 6' draught x 9'6" air draught, must represent something approaching the absolute maximum for any craft attempting to negotiate the waterways described here (especially with regard to combined keel and air draught). Indeed, some of the cruising grounds were in fact denied to *Valcon* (the River Derwent and the Pocklington Canal to name but two) but the list of recommended reading offers specialist information, from specialised authorities all of whom have been extremely generous with their time and help; so when it comes to the very last drying-out, no-longer-working locked pound, there will always be a word from those with the local knowledge to be able specially to plead its cause.

This, then, is an appropriate place to mention that much of the factual and 'official' information was unearthed, tabulated or confirmed by the official authorities, boards and services in the area as well the clubs, organisations and many, many individuals who were all committed to getting the facts right and the record straight. The section that follows is a tribute to their assiduousness, conscientiousness and general willingness to help.

TABLE OF DISTANCES – MAIN ROUTES

	Bawtry	Beverley	Boston	Brigg	Goole (Canal)	Goole (River)	Hull	Leeds	Lincoln	Newark	Nottingham	Pocklington	Ripon	Selby (Canal)	Selby (River)	Sheffield	Sowerby Bridge	Stamford Bridge	Wakefield	Worksop	York
Bawtry		58	68	52	55	41	48	70	36	50	70	70	100	65	57	65	90	70	70	37	76
Beverley	58		105	26		33	10	67	75	83	103	62	92	75	49	77	85	62	65	57	60
Boston	68	105		100	97	88	95	117	32	65	85	117	150	113	103	110	135	117	115	83	123
Brigg	52	26	100			28	16	62	100	77	97	57	90		44	71	80	57	60	78	118
Goole (Canal)	55		97					34	64	75	95			28		40	51		31	65	
Goole (River)	41	33	88	28			23		55	65	85	30	60		15	58		30		55	33
Hull	48	10	95	16		23		57	63	74	94	52	82	43	38	66	74	53	54	62	56
Leeds	70	67	117	62	34		57		82	92	112	55	75	29	49	60	38	55	18	84	47
Lincoln	36	75	32	100	64	55	63	82		34	54	84	128	78	71	80	100	84	80	52	100
Newark	50	83	65	77	75	65	74	92	34		20	92	125	88	80	90	110	92	90	62	98
Nottingham	70	103	85	97	95	85	94	112	54	20		112	145	108	100	110	130	112	110	82	118
Pocklington	70	62	117	57		30	52	55	84	92	112		72		26	63	80	20	60	84	44
Ripon	100	92	150	90		60	82	75	128	125	145	72			45	100	92	71	72	120	27
Selby (Canal)	65	75	113		28		43	29	78	88	108					53	46		26	78	
Selby (River)	57	49	103	44		15	38	49	71	80	100	26	45			55	66	26	46	70	46
Sheffield	65	77	110	71	40	58	66	60	80	90	110	63	100	53	55		77	69	57	80	74
Sowerby Bridge	90	85	135	80	51		74	38	100	110	130	80	92	46	66	77		70	20	100	65
Stamford Bridge	70	62	117	57		30	53	55	84	92	112	20	71		26	69	70		50	86	44
Wakefield	70	65	115	60	31		54	18	80	90	110	60	72	26	46	57	20	50		80	45
Worksop	37	57	83	78	65	55	62	84	52	62	82	84	120	78	70	80	100	86	80		68
York	76	60	123	118		33	56	47	100	98	118	44	27		46	74	65	44	45	68	

	Miles	Locks		Miles	Locks
Witham & Fossdyke			**Calder & Hebble**	21	25
River Witham	30	3	Selby Canal	12	4
Fossdyke	10	1			
			Ouse		
Trent			River Ouse	60	1
River Trent	80	7	River Ure	7	2
River Idle	10	1	Ripon Canal	1	1
Chesterfield Canal	25	16	River Derwent	25	1
			Pocklington Canal	10	8
Sheffield & South Yorkshire					
Sheffield & S. Yorkshire	28	24	**Ancholme & Hull**		
Stainforth & Keadby	14	3	River Ancholme	13	1
New Junction Canal	6	1	River Hull	15	—
Aire & Calder Navigation					
Goole to Castleford	24	6			
Castleford to Leeds	10	5			
Castleford to Wakefield	7	5			

For comprehensive distance tables see L. A. Edwards. *Inland Waterways of Great Britain*. Imray 1985.

AUTHORITIES

I. The Witham & Fossdyke

Navigation authority
British Waterways Board,
24 Meadow Lane,
Nottingham NG2 3HL
☎ (0602) 862411

Water authority
Anglian Water,
Waterside House,
Waterside North,
Lincoln LN2 5HA
☎ (0522) 25231

Northern Area Office,
Guy Gibson Hall,
Manby Park,
Louth LN11 8UR
☎ (050 782) 8101

Southern Area Office,
Aqua House,
Harvey Street,
Lincoln LN1 1TF
☎ (0522) 39221

**Witham Fourth District Internal
Drainage Board,**
47 Norfolk Street,
Boston, Lincs.
(for Witham Navigable Drains)

II. The Trent

Navigation authority
British Waterways Board,
24 Meadow Lane,
Nottingham NG2 3HL
☎ (0602) 862411

This is the licensing authority for the river between Shardlow and Gainsborough.

Associated British Ports (Hull),
Kingston House Tower,
Bond Street,
Hull HU1 3ER
☎ (0482) 27171

This is the navigation authority up to the South side of the Stone Bridge in Gainsborough. No licence is required.

Water authority
Severn-Trent Water Authority,
Lower Trent Division,
Mapperley Hall,
Lucknow Avenue,
Nottingham NG3 5BN
☎ (0602) 608161

III. The Sheffield & South Yorkshire Canal

Navigation authority
British Waterways Board,
(Castleford Area),
Lock Lane,
Castleford WF10 2LH
☎ (0977) 554351/5
After hours 554351 connects with Securicor Bradford for emergency use.

Water authority
Yorkshire Water,
21 Park Square South,
Leeds LS1 2QG
☎ (0532) 440191

IV. The Aire & Calder

British Waterways Board,
(Castleford Area),
Lock Lane,
Castleford WF10 2LH
☎ (0977) 554351/5

Water authority
Yorkshire Water,
21 Park Square South,
Leeds LS1 2QG.
☎ (0532) 440191

V. The Ouse

Navigation authority
Associated British Ports (Hull),
Kingston House Tower,
Bond Street,
Hull HU1 3ER
☎(0482) 27171

(From Trent Falls to a point 100 yards below the Hook Railway Bridge.)

The Ouse Navigation Trustees,
7 St. Leonard's Place,
York YO1 2EU
Captain Rimmer, Naburn Locks
☎ (090487) 229 or 258
(From the above to 2 miles below Linton Lock)

Linton Lock Commissioners
1/3 Wheelgate,
Malton, Yorkshire.

(From the above to source.)

British Waterways Board,
Castleford Area,
Lock Lane,
Castleford, WF10 2LH
☎ (0977) 554351/5
(For the River Ure, the Ripon Canal and the
Pocklington Canal)

Water authority
Yorkshire Water,
21 Park Square South,
Leeds LS1 2QG
☎ (0532) 440191
(For River Derwent)

VI. The Ancholme and the Hull

The River Ancholme

Anglian Water,
Waterside House,
Waterside North,
Lincoln LN2 5HA
☎ (0522) 25231

AW office and lock-keeper,
South Ferriby
☎ (0652) 635219
VHF channels 16, 06, 10, 12, 14

Northern Area Office,
Guy Gibson Hall,
Manby Park,
Louth LN11 8UR
☎ (050 782) 8101

Southern Area Office,
Aqua House,
Harvey Street,
Lincoln LN1 1TF
☎ (0522) 39221

The River Hull

Navigation authority
Hull City Council,
Engineer's Department,
Guildhall,
Alfred Gelder Street,
Hull HU1 2AA
☎ (0482) 223111

Harbour master
Drypool Bridge
☎ (0482) 222287
VHF channels 16 and 12 for three hours befc
and one hour after HW.

Water authority
Yorkshire Water Authority
Head Office,
West Riding House,
67 Albion Street,
Leeds LS1 5AA
☎ (0532) 448201

Rivers Division,
21 Park Square South,
Leeds LS1 2QG
☎ (0532) 440191

North & East Division,
Monkgate,
York
☎ (0482) 27171

The River Humber

Associated British Ports (Hull)
Kingston House Tower,
Bond Street,
Hull HU1 3ER
☎ (0482) 701787

Associated British Ports

Goole
The Port Manager,
Dock Offices, Stanhope Street,
Goole,
North Humberside
☎ (0405) 2691

Hull
The Port Manager,
P.O. Box 1,
Kingston House Tower,
Bond Street,
Hull HU1 3ER
☎ (0482) 27171

Grimsby
The Port Manager,
Grimsby,
South Humberside DN31 3LL
☎ (0472) 59181

Immingham
The Docks Manager,
Dock Office,
Immingham
☎ (0469) 73441

British Waterways Board

Northern Region Office
1 Dock Street,
Leeds LS1 1HH
☎ (0532) 436741

Head Office
Melbury House,
Melbury Terrace,
London NW1 6JX
☎ 01 262 6711

BWB Canalphone
(for unscheduled stoppages)
☎ 01 723 8486

Key to Symbols used on the plans

	☎ Telephone	Sanitary Station	⚓ Short Stay Mooring	
⚓ Water	✉ Post Office	W.C.	● Gas	
Fuel	Repairs	Public House		
S Shops	Shower	✕ Restaurant		

In the notes on locks and bridges
● means that the lock/bridge is operated in the way described.

TIDAL DIFFERENCES ON HIGH WATER IMMINGHAM
(Humber, Ouse and Trent)

| | High water | | Flood | | Duration of rises | |
	Neaps	Springs	Neaps	Springs	Neaps	Springs
River Humber	*hr. m.*	*hr. m.*	*hr. m.*	*hr. m.*	*hr. m.*	*hr. m.*
Spurn	− 0 15	0 15	− 6 45	6 18	6 30	6 03
Grimsby	− 0 05	0 09	− 6 25	6 09	6 20	6 00
Immingham	0	0	− 6 20	5 53	6 20	5 53
Hull	+ 0 21	0 20	− 5 50	5 15	6 11	5 35
Hessle	+ 0 35	0 30	− 5 20	4 45	5 55	5 15
Ferriby Sluice	+ 0 40	0 35	− 4 50	4 15	5 30	4 50
Trent Falls	+ 1 00	0 50	− 3 20	2 50	4 20	3 40
Blacktoft	+ 1 05	0 55	− 3 05	2 35	4 10	3 30
Goole	+ 1 30	1 15	− 2 30	2 00	4 00	3 15
Bramby	+ 2 00	1 30	− 1 45	1 15	3 45	2 45
Selby	+ 2 30	2 00	− 0 15	+ 0 15	2 45	1 45
Cawood	+ 3 35	2 45	+ 1 15	1 30	2 20	1 15
Naburn	+ 4 30	3 30	+ 2 30	2 00	2 00	1 30
River Trent						
Keadby	+ 1 30	1 15	− 2 15	1 45	3 45	3 00
West Stockwith	+ 2 20	1 50	− 0 50	0 15	3 10	2 05
Gainsborough	+ 2 15	2 45	− 0 20	+ 0 20	3 05	1 55
Torksey	+ 3 45	3 40	+ 1 10	1 45	2 35	1 55
Cromwell	+ 5 00		+ 4 00		1 00	

BRITISH WATERWAYS BOARD CODE OF CONDUCT

Sound signals

One Short Blast (about 1 second)	I'm altering my course to starboard (to the right)
Two Short Blasts	I'm altering my course to port (to the left)
Three Short Blasts	My engine is going astern (in reverse)
Four Short Blasts	I'm about to manoeuvre (always followed by one or two short blasts as above)
One Long Blast	To be sounded every 20 seconds when approaching a bend

Rules of the road

On inland waterways always keep to the **right** when passing a boat coming from the opposite direction.

If you overtake another boat you do so on the **left** and at a slow speed.

Do **not** overtake on a bend, near a bridge, lock or when you cannot see a clear way ahead.

When being overtaken by another boat slow down so as to just have steerage way.

You usually find deeper water on the outside of bends, but look out for other craft.

Pleasure craft should keep well clear upstream or downstream of commercial craft whilst they are manoeuvring at wharves, staithes, in locks etc. Watch out for sea-going vessels, they have limited manoeuvrability.

If you meet a deep-draughted boat which has to hug the outside of the bend pass on the **left**.

Remember sailing boats cannot manoeuvre as easily as powered craft. On rivers where sailing boats may be found, powered boats should try to keep clear. When overtaking or meeting a sailing boat when it is tacking, always pass under its stern or watch for guidance from the skipper.

If it is not possible to pass on the right e.g. when a boat is being towed from the towing path, pass on the 'wrong' side, the **left**.

Sound your horn twice to let the other boat know.

Slow down before you reach bends, bridges locks, tunnels or repair works.

Speed limits

Observe speed limits at all times, never go faster except where it is **essential** to your safety in tidal or flooding waters.

4 miles per hour – is the limit on most inland waterways. This is about a fast walking pace.

Certain river navigations have different speed limits which are as follows:

6 miles per hour upstream, 8 miles per hour downstream – The Trent Navigation (except between Averham Weir and Newark Nether Lock and between Beeston Lock and Meadow Lane Lock, Nottingham, 4 mph).

6 miles per hour – Aire and Calder Navigation (except the Selby Canal), the New Junction Canal, Sheffield and South Yorkshire Navigation, and Witham Navigation.

Where water ski-ing is in progress, this will be at specified zones and only club members are allowed to exceed the speed limit.

Sometimes set speed limits are too fast for the water conditions. You will know this because the wash of the boat is breaking like waves on a beach. If it does this slow down at once. Bow or stern waves indicate that you are likely to be using more fuel than you need. The waves which you are creating also cause a nuisance to other waterway users, particularly fishermen and moored boats. The waves cause extensive damage to the banks and can also cause physical damage to moored boats.

In shallow water your boat will actually travel faster if you reduce engine speed as over-revving pulls the bottom of the boat deep into the mud.

When you are passing fishermen, moored boats and small unpowered craft such as rowing boats reduce speed to a level at which disturbance is negligible.

Tying up

On river navigations it is suggested that you moor with the bow of your boat facing upstream. On tidal waters, moor with the bow facing the tide. Never tie your ropes across the towing path; use rings or bollards as provided or hammer your stakes on the canalside of the path.

Usually the bank opposite the towing path is private property. On river navigations both banks are often private property.

Where possible boats should moor at approved temporary mooring places where facilities for rubbish disposal, etc. can often be found.

If you do moor against the towing path, due regard should be given to anglers and other users of the towing path.

Always moor in a position where your boat is not a hazard to navigation. A boat must be tied up at the bow and stern.

Try to avoid mooring overnight on tidal waters.

Never moor longer than necessary at water points or sanitary disposal stations. Move away as soon as possible to allow others access to facilities.

Do not moor by 'blind' bridges, in lock entrances or near sharp bends and junctions – you might be rammed!

Do not moor on the outside of bends. That wall may look inviting, but large boats need the channel on the outside of bends.

Angling

Watch out for fishermen. At fishing matches there is often warning given by a notice erected on the towing paths. Please slow down and keep to the centre of the channel.

Lift and swing bridges

Before setting out make sure that you know **exactly** how to operate lift and swing bridges.

Children should **never** be allowed to operate lift and swing bridges. There should always be an adult on board the boat, do not leave children alone when navigating a swing or lift bridge. Particular care should be taken to ensure adequate clearances between the boat, the crew on board and bridge structures.

Extra care **must** be taken when operating these bridges.

Tunnels

Do not enter the tunnel until it is clear. Switch on headlight and sound hooter. Look out for unpowered craft.

Proceed at a moderate speed and beware of water dripping from the roof. Never enter a tunnel without making sure that your boat is equipped with adequate lights and ensure nobody is standing on the cabin side or roof.

Users of unpowered boats are not allowed in some tunnels, and in some others only under certain conditions.

Rivers

Boaters are reminded that rivers have a faster flow than canals and some are tidal. Extra care should be taken on rivers particularly when wind or flow conditions are such that navigation is made hazardous. If you are on a river that is flooding make sure that any predicted rises will not stop you navigating under bridges and if the boat is moored the ropes must have plenty of scope to allow for the rise and fall of water level, especially if you are moored overnight.

Under no circumstances go on a river when there is any flood water about without a sufficiently heavy anchor and a strong cable or anchor rope at least five times as long as the deepest part of the river. It is vital that there is a strong anchorage point for making the cable fast to.

You should also have on board life-buoys, etc. with lines on for emergency use. All boats should be kept well away from weirs.

Keep a good look-out for floating debris, such as tree trunks, which could sink or over-turn a small boat.

Towing paths

Care must be taken not to obstruct the towing path or leave anything in such a way that people could trip over it. It is easy to see the path that people will be following.

Similarly, boats should be moored without lines or pins obstructing the towing path.

Locks

The British Waterways Board continue to ask for the co-operation of all users of the Board's cruising and remainder waterways by not using the locks during the hours of darkness (extending from lighting-up time to sunrise). However, it will be necessary to continue more severe restrictions on some structures and certain locks at critical points, where any incorrect operation could cause flooding and danger to public safety or where the drainage of a major pound would cause serious interruption to cruising.

British Waterways Board wish to trust the boater not to use the locks at night.

The standard windlass with two tapered apertures measuring 1″ and 1¼″ respectively can usually be purchased during normal hours from many of the Board's offices, including Castleford, Nottingham and Leeds. In addition, windlasses are obtainable from many boatyards.

For the Calder and Hebble Navigation from Shepley Bridge to Sowerby Bridge hand spikes are required and these may be obtained during normal working hours from either the area office at Castleford or section office at Shepley Bridge, Huddersfield Road, Mirfield.

Visitors to the Ripon Canal are advised that Oxclose Lock is padlocked at most times, in order to deter vandalism. However, keys are available at the area office at Castleford and at Selby Lock. Boat users are requested to leave Oxclose Lock as they found it.

Boat users are reminded how essential it is to ensure that lock gates and paddles are fully closed after use.

It is necessary to institute emergency and additional stoppages according to local circumstances and before cruising, you are advised to telephone Canalphone 01 723 8486 for the latest situation or contact your local area office.

Make sure you know exactly how to work a lock before you enter one.

Do not attempt to use staircase locks until you know the correct procedure.

Check the following:

That your boat is completely inside the lock.

When going uphill your rudder cannot catch in the bottom gates.

When going downhill make sure that the rear of the boat is not likely to sit on the sill.

That nobody is standing on the roof or foredeck when entering a lock, the bump of the boat against the side may throw them in.

Do not leave windlasses on spindles as they could fly off if the paddles are run down.

Be careful not to trap your fingers in any of the mechanisms, or between ropes and bollards.

Never assume that the previous boat has left the lock mechanisms correctly.

In narrow locks be aware that a boat tends to be drawn to the upper gate when the lock is filling.

Do not use a lock in the dark, it is only too easy for someone to fall into the water and not be heard or seen.

Do not let anyone play near locks, be it running around or jumping over gates etc. It is not worth the risk of them falling in.

You should know exactly what to do if someone falls into the water. If this happens close all the paddles immediately and throw them a lifebuoy. Then consider how to get them out – possibly this could be done by filling the lock up slowly to bring them to your level.

Never dangle your arms or legs over the side of the boat, they may get broken or crushed between the boat and the lock.

Beware of floating debris between the boat and the lock.

Going up

1 Make sure the top gates and paddles are closed.

2 If lock is full, empty it by raising bottom paddles.

3 Open bottom gates and enter lock.

4 Close bottom gates behind you and lower the paddles.

5 Open the top paddles to fill lock.

6 Open top gates and take your boat out.

7 Close gates behind you and lower the paddles.

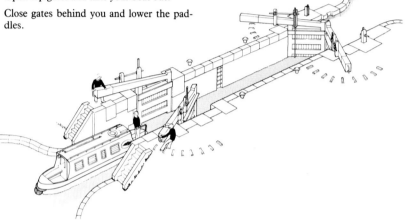

Operating locks is simple if you work through the drill systematically, and *never* hurry.

Always share a lock with other boats (this saves water supplies) and wait turns whenever possible.

Secure boat in lock by looping ropes round the bollards provided.

Do not tie.

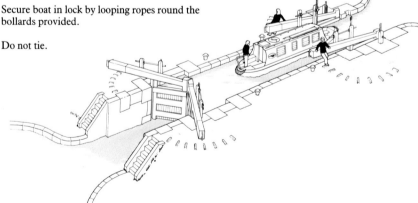

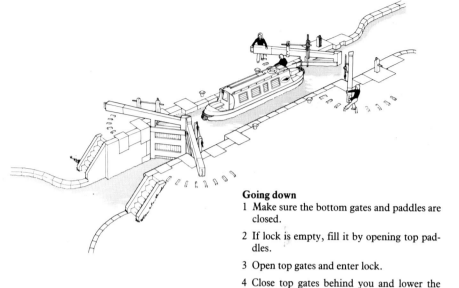

Going down

1 Make sure the bottom gates and paddles are closed.

2 If lock is empty, fill it by opening top paddles.

3 Open top gates and enter lock.

4 Close top gates behind you and lower the paddles.

5 Open bottom paddles to empty lock.

6 Open bottom gates and take your boat out.

7 Close gates behind you and lower paddles.

Always ensure that all gates and paddles are closed after you leave the lock.

It is better to wait a few minutes and share the lock with another boat than to close the gates on an approaching boat and waste 20,000 gallons of water (or more).

PUMP OUT LOCATIONS

Fossdyke & Witham Navigations
Lincoln – Brayford Trust

Trent Navigation
Fiskerton – Fiskerton Wharf

SANITARY STATIONS 🚽

Many sanitary disposal stations are now open and keys may be bought from the majority of boat yards and boat clubs as well as from the Board's office. This key may also be required to gain access to water points.

Aire & Calder Navigation
Whitley Bridge – Whitley Lock
Castleford Junction – Castleford Lock
Leeds – Leeds Lock
Goole – Alongside Smith Bros.

Calder & Hebble Navigation
Wakefield – BWB Freight Depot
Dewsbury – Savile Town Basin, Robinson's Hire Cruisers
Shepley Bridge – Shepley Bridge, BWB Maintenance Yard
Brighouse – Brighouse Basin
Salterhebble Lock

Selby Canal
Selby – Selby Basin

Sheffield & South Yorkshire Navigation
Keadby – Keadby Lock
Thorne – BWB Maintenance Yard
Swinton – Waddington Lock

River Ure Navigation
Boroughbridge – The Wharf

Chesterfield Canal
West Stockwith – West Stockwith Yacht Basin Clayworth
Worksop – BWB Maintenance Yard

Fossdyke & Witham Navigations
Torksey – Torksey Lock
Lincoln – BWB Maintenance Yard
Lincoln – Brayford Trust
Bardney – Shortferry Marina
Dogdyke – Belle Isle Boat Hire
Boston – Grand Sluice Lock

Trent Navigation
Nottingham – Meadow Lane Lock
Nottingham – Park Yacht Club
Colwick – Colwick Marina
Gunthorpe – Gunthorpe Lock
Fiskerton – Fiskerton Wharf
Farndon – Farndon Harbour
Newark – Newark Town Lock
Newark – Newark Nether Lock

BWB WATER POINTS 🚰

Aire & Calder Navigation
Stanley Ferry – Between Stanley Ferry Aqueduct and Ramsden's Swing Bridge
Altofts – King's Road Lock
Altofts – Woodnock Lock
Beal – Beal Lock
Goole – The Timber Pond, Smith Bros.
Pollington – No 3 Swing Bridge
Great Heck – Heck, South Yorkshire Boat Club
Whitley Bridge – Whitley Lock
Ferrybridge – Ferrybridge Lock
Castleford Junction – Castleford Lock
Allerton Bywater – Kippax Lock
Woodlesford – Woodlesford Lock
Leeds – Fishpond Lock
Leeds – Leeds Lock

Calder & Hebble Navigation
Wakefield – Wakefield Flood Lock
Wakefield – West Riding Marine
Horbury – Broad Cut Low Lock
Thornhill – Figure of Three Locks
Dewsbury – Savile Town Basin, Robinson's Hire Cruisers
Dewsbury – Double Locks
Mirfield – Shepley Bridge, BWB Maintenance Yard
Mirfield – Yorkshire Motor Yachts
Brighouse – Brighouse Basin
Halifax – Salterhebble Locks
Sowerby Bridge – Shire Cruisers

Huddersfield Broad Canal
Huddersfield

Selby Canal
Selby – Selby Lock

Sheffield & South Yorkshire Navigation
Keadby – Keadby Lock
Keadby – Keadby Marine
Thorne – BWB Maintenance Yard

Thorne – Ladyline
Thorne – Stanilands Marina
Thorne – Blue Water Marina
Doncaster – Long Sandall Lock
Doncaster – Strawberry Island Boat Club
Sprotbrough – Sprotbrough Lock
Mexborough – Mexborough Low Lock
Mexborough – Mexborough Top Lock
Swinton – Waddington Lock
Kilnhurst – Kilnhurst Lock
Rotherham – Aldwarke Lock
Rotherham – Frank Price Lock
Sheffield – Sheffield Basin

Chesterfield Canal
West Stockwith – West Stockwith Yacht Basin
Drakeholes
Claywood
Retford – Retford Marina
Retford – Forest Locks
Worksop – BWB Maintenance Yard

Fossdyke & Witham Navigations
Torksey – Torksey Lock
Lincoln – BWB Maintenance Yard
Lincoln – Brayford Trust
Lincoln – Stamp End Lock
Bardney – Bardney Bridge
Bardney – Shortferry Marina

Dogdyke – Belle Isle Boat Hire
Boston – Grand Sluice Lock
Boston – Boston Marina

Trent Navigation
Nottingham – Trevithicks Boatyard
Nottingham – Castle Marina
Nottingham – Meadow Lane Marina
Nottingham – Speed Electrics
Nottingham – Park Yacht Club
Colwick – Colwick Marine
Holme – Holme Lock
Stoke Bardolph – Stoke Bardolph Lock
East Bridgford – East Bridgford Marine
Gunthorpe – Damark Marine
Gunthorpe – Gunthorpe Lock
Bleasby – Hazleford Lock
Fiskerton – Fiskerton Wharf
Farndon – Farndon Ferry
Farndon – Farndon Harbour
Newark – Newark Marina
Newark – Newark Town Lock
Newark – Newark Nether Lock
Cromwell – Cromwell Lock

VHF RADIO AT LOCKS

The following locks in the area are equipped
with Marine Band VHF radios.

| | | | Channels | |
Lock	Call Sign	Set	Watch	Working
Cromwell	Cromwell Lock	Fixed	16+ 74	74
Newark Nether	Nether Lock	Fixed	16+ 74	74
Newark Town	Town Lock	Fixed	16+ 74	74
Hazleford	Hazleford Lock	Fixed	16+ 74	74
Gunthorpe	Gunthorpe Lock	Fixed	16+ 74	74
Stoke Bardolph	Stoke Lock	Fixed	16+ 74	74
Holme	Holme Lock	Fixed	16+ 74	74
Torksey	Torksey Lock	Fixed	16+ 74	74
West Stockwith	Stockwith Lock	Fixed	16+ 74	74
Boston	Grand Sluice Lock	Portable	16	74
Keadby	Keadby Lock	Fixed	16+ 74	74

The system is for communication between
locks and between craft and locks with the
object of assisting in the safe passage of craft.

The lock-keeper will, if requested, inform the
next lock of intended passage. If, however, a
craft decides not to complete the journey but to
stop for a period at an intermediate location the
boater is requested to please inform the next
lock.

PLEASURE BOAT LICENCES AND REGISTRATION CERTIFICATES

Pleasure boat licences are required for privately owned pleasure boats on the Board's waterways. They allow the boat to be on the waterways that are available for pleasure cruising, including the Board's river waterways. They are issued subject to Conditions, and do not permit you to hire the boat to others.

River registration certificates are required for pleasure boats on the Board's river waterways only (including the Trent, Fossdyke and Witham, and Ure), and are not valid on the canals.

Licences and certificates are available for 12, 6, 3 and 1 months and 7 days. Further details are available from the area offices or the Craft Licensing Office, Willow Grange, Church Road, Watford.

An information circular is issued twice yearly by the Board. This gives details of opening times of manned locks and bridges, telephone numbers of tidal locks and VHF channels where installed.

RECOMMENDED READING

BOOKS

Cruising Guide to the North East Waterways
    Published by the Ripon Motor Boat Club and available from:
    Frank Ryan, esq., Acting honorary secretary, 95 Harlow Crescent, Harrogate HG2 0AL

A Guide to the Pocklington Canal
    Published by the Pocklington Canal Amenity Society and available from:
    Mrs. S. M. Nix, 74 Westminster Road, York YO3 6LY
    ☎ York (0904) 23338

The Derwent Guide
    Published by the Yorkshire Derwent Trust and available from:
    R. I. Womersley, esq., 25 Cloverley Drive, Timperley, Altrincham, Cheshire
    ☎ Manchester (061) 980 3478

A Guide to the Driffield Navigation
    Published jointly by Commissioners of the Driffield Navigation and Driffield Navigation Amenities Association, and available from:
    Alan Ball, esq., 12 Weighton Grove, Hull
    ☎ Hull (0482) 442884

The Chesterfield Canal (West Stockwith to Rhodesia)
    Published by the Chesterfield Canal Society and available from:
    Chris Richardson, 15 Coral Drive, Aughton, Sheffield S31 0RA
    ☎ Sheffield (0742) 874537

West Yorkshire Waterway Guide. Calder Navigation Society. Available from:
    Keith Noble, The Dene, Triangle, Sowerby Bridge, W. Yorks HX6 3EA
    ☎ Halifax (0422) 823562

Planning a Trip on the Ouse, Trent and Humber
    Published by and available from the author:
    J. A. Hutton, Esq., 121 The Meadows, Cherry Burton, Beverley
    ☎ Leconfield (0401) 50877

The Tidal Havens of the Wash and Humber
    Henry Irving. Imray, Laurie, Norie & Wilson 1983.

Inland Waterways of Great Britain
    L. A. Edwards. Imray, Laurie, Norie & Wilson 1985.

CHARTS
Tidal Ouse – Tidal Trent – Non-tidal Trent
 Published by the Trent Boating Association and available from:
 Tom Pattison, esq., 16 Baker Avenue, Arnold, Notts. NG5 8FU
 ☎ Nottingham (0602) 262055

MAPS
Lockmaster Nos 4 and 7: South Yorkshire's Waterways; Nottinghamshire's Waterways
 Published by and available from the originator:
 Douglas B. Smith, Esq., Kingswood Cottage, Dicks Lane Wharf, Rowington,
 Warwick CB35 7DN
 ☎ Lapworth (05643) 3233

Map of the Inland Waterways of England and Wales.
 Imray, Laurie, Norie and Wilson.

ORDNANCE SURVEY
EAST MIDLANDS AND YORKSHIRE
1:250 000 Routemaster 6.

THE WITHAM AND THE FOSSDYKE
1:50 000 Landranger. 131 Boston & Spalding. 122 Skegness. 121 Lincoln.

THE TRENT
1:50 000 Landranger. 112 Scunthorpe. 120 Mansfield and the Dukeries. 129 Nottingham and Loughborough.

THE SHEFFIELD & SOUTH YORKSHIRE NAVIGATION
1:50 000 Landranger. 112 Scunthorpe. 111 Doncaster.

THE AIRE & CALDER NAVIGATION
1:50 000 Landranger. 104 Leeds and Bradford. 105 York. 111 Sheffield and Doncaster. 110 Sheffield and Huddersfield.

THE YORKSHIRE OUSE
1:50 000 Landranger. 105 York. 99 Northallerton and Ripon. 100 Malton and Pickering.

THE ANCHOLME AND THE HULL
1:50 000 Landranger. 112 Scunthorpe (for the Ancholme). 107 Kingston upon Hull (for the Hull). Both can be used for the Humber.

WHARVES IN USE FOR FREIGHT ON NORTHEAST WATERWAYS

The following information was compiled by John Pomfret of the NE. ISC. Section of the Inland Waterways Association. He can be contacted at 8 Hillcrest, Durham DH1 1RB.

In general, wharves on the Humber, Trent up to Gainsborough, Ouse up to Selby and at Goole are principally used by coasters. The River Hull is a mixture. Other wharves are served by dry cargo or tanker barges as appropriate. Of particular note are the Tom Puddings, which operate with coke from Doncaster to Goole and the Cawood -Hargreaves 'pans', which operate from the five coal staithes to Ferrybridge 'C' Power Station.

KEY TO TABLES
The numbers appearing in the left-hand column can be located on the accompanying map of 'Wharves used Commercially'. There are large-scale maps for the Castleford/Knottingley, Selby and York areas.

17

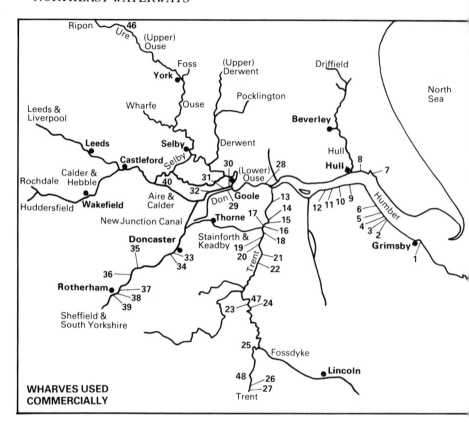

**WHARVES USED
COMMERCIALLY**

KEY TO MAP SHOWING WHARVES IN USE FOR FREIGHT

Name of wharf and authority (user)	*Trade*
HUMBER	
1 Grimsby Docks – ABP	General
2 Immingham Oil Terminal – APT	Petroleum
3 Immingham Docks – ABP	General
4 Immingham Bulk Terminal – NCB/BSC	Ore, coal
5 South Killingholme Oil Jetty – Texaco	Petroleum
6 North Killingholme Oil Jetty – Shell	Petroleum
7 Saltend Oil Terminal – BP	Petroleum
8 King George V Dock, Hull – ABP	General
9 New Holland Basin – Howarth	Timber, scrap
9 New Holland Pier – GEM	Bulks
10 Barrow Haven – Humberbank	General
11 Barrow Clayfields – Foster	General
12 Barton Haven – Albright & Wilson	Chemicals

Name of wharf and authority (user)	*Trade*
TRENT	
13 Burton Stather – Kingsferry Wharf	General
14 Flixborough – BSC consortium	Ore, steel, coal
15 Neap House – LSD	General
16 Grove Wharf – Wharton Shipping	General
17 Keadby Wharf – Wharton Shipping	General
18 Gunness Wharf – Gunness Wharf	General
19 Althorpe Wharf – Gunness Wharf	General
20 Derrythorpe Layby Jetty – ABP	—
21 Butterwick Layby Jetty – ABP	—
22 Messingham Wharf – British Industrial Sand	Glass sand
23 Beckingham – Trent Wharfage	Ore, animal feed
24 Gainsborough – BWB	General
– Whitton & Curtis Moody	Cereals
47 Reeves – Millgate	Cement, general
25 Rampton (Cottam) – Steetley Construction	Aggregates
48 High Marnham Power Station – CEGB	Fuel oil
26 Girton – Hoveringham Gravels	Aggregates
27 Besthorpe – Redland Aggregates	Aggregates
LOWER OUSE/DUTCH RIVER	
28 Blacktoft Layby Jetty – ABP	—
29 Fisons Wharf – Fisons	Fertilizers
30 Goole Docks – ABP	General
AIRE & CALDER NAVIGATION	
31 Goole BWB – BWB	General
32 Rawcliffe Bridge – BWB/Croda	Oil seeds & nuts
SOUTH YORKSHIRE CANAL	
33 Gas House, Doncaster – Waddington	Steel
34 Doncaster Depot – BWB	Coke
35 Swinton – Waddington	Steel
36 Kilnhurst – Croda	Black oil, pitch
37 Eastwood – Waddington	Steel
38 Eastwood – Sheffield Haulage/Storage :	Steel
39 Rawmarsh, Rotherham – BWB	General
AIRE & CALDER NAVIGATION	
40 Whitley Bridge – BWB/BOCM	Animal feeds
41 Stanley Ferry	
42 Wakefield Oil Wharf – British Fuel Co	Petroleum
43 Knostrop Depot, Leeds – BWB	General
44 Petrofina Wharf	Petroleum

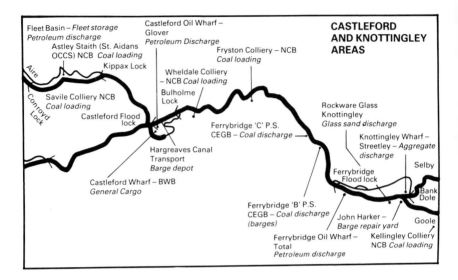

OUSE & FOSS

See plan for detail of York Area.

45 Howdendyke – Humberside Sea & Land   Fertilizers etc.
46 Boroughbridge – R W Potter   Aggregates

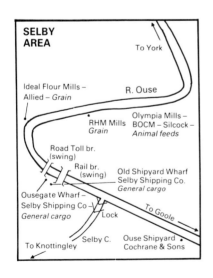

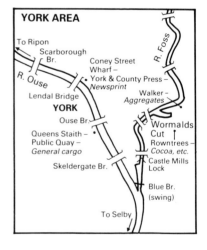

CONVERSION TABLES

ENGLISH MILES TO KILOMETRES (100 miles = 160.93 kilometres)

Miles	0	10	20	30	40	50	60	70	80	90
0	Kilometres 16.09	32.19	48.28	64.37	80.47	96.56	112.65	128.75	144.84
1	1.61	17.70	33.80	49.89	65.98	82.08	98.17	114.26	130.36	146.45
2	3.22	19.31	35.41	51.50	67.59	83.69	99.78	115.87	131.97	148.06
3	4.83	20.92	37.01	53.11	69.20	85.29	101.39	117.48	133.58	149.67
4	6.44	22.53	38.62	54.72	70.81	86.90	103.00	119.09	135.18	151.28
5	8.05	24.14	40.23	56.33	72.42	88.51	104.61	120.70	136.79	152.89
6	9.66	25.75	41.84	57.94	74.03	90.12	106.22	122.31	138.40	154.50
7	11.26	27.36	43.45	59.55	75.64	91.73	107.83	123.92	140.01	156.11
8	12.87	28.97	45.06	61.15	77.25	93.34	109.44	125.53	141.62	157.72
9	13.48	30.58	46.67	62.76	78.86	94.95	111.04	127.14	143.23	159.32

KILOMETRES TO ENGLISH MILES (100 kilometres = 62.137 miles)

Kilometres	0	10	20	30	40	50	60	70	80	90
0	Miles 6.21	12.43	18.64	24.85	31.07	37.28	43.50	49.71	55.92
1	0.62	6.83	13.05	19.26	25.48	31.70	37.90	44.12	50.33	56.54
2	1.24	7.46	13.67	19.88	26.10	32.31	38.52	44.74	50.95	57.17
3	1.86	8.08	14.29	20.50	26.72	32.93	39.15	45.36	51.57	57.79
4	2.48	8.70	14.91	21.13	27.34	33.55	39.77	45.98	52.19	58.41
5	3.11	9.32	15.53	21.75	27.96	34.17	40.39	46.60	52.82	59.03
6	3.73	9.94	16.16	22.37	28.58	34.80	41.01	47.22	53.44	59.65
7	4.35	10.56	16.78	22.99	29.20	35.42	41.63	47.85	54.06	60.27
8	4.97	11.18	17.40	23.61	29.83	36.04	42.25	48.47	54.68	60.89
9	5.59	11.81	18.02	24.23	30.45	36.66	42.87	49.09	55.30	61.52

ENGLISH FEET TO METRES (100 kilometres = 30.479 metres)

Feet	0	10	20	30	40	50	60	70	80	90
0	Metres 3.05	6.03	9.14	12.19	15.24	18.29	21.33	24.38	27.43
1	0.30	3.35	6.40	9.44	12.50	15.54	18.59	21.64	24.69	27.74
2	0.61	3.66	6.70	9.75	12.80	15.85	18.90	21.94	24.99	28.04
3	0.91	3.96	7.01	10.06	13.11	16.15	19.20	22.25	25.30	28.35
4	1.22	4.28	7.31	10.36	13.41	16.46	19.51	22.55	25.60	28.65
5	1.52	4.57	7.62	10.67	13.72	16.76	19.81	22.86	25.91	28.95
6	1.83	4.88	7.92	10.97	14.02	17.07	20.12	23.16	26.21	29.26
7	2.13	5.18	8.23	11.28	14.32	17.37	20.42	23.47	26.52	29.56
8	2.44	5.49	8.53	11.58	14.63	17.68	20.73	23.77	26.82	29.87
9	2.74	5.79	8.84	11.89	14.93	17.98	21.03	24.08	27.13	30.17

METRES TO ENGLISH FEET (100 kilometres = 328.09 feet)

Metres	0	10	20	30	40	50	60	70	80	90
0	Feet	32.8	65.6	98.4	131.2	164.0	196.8	229.7	262.5	295.3
1	3.3	36.1	68.9	101.7	134.5	167.3	200.1	232.9	265.7	298.6
2	6.6	39.4	72.2	105.0	137.8	170.6	203.4	236.2	269.0	301.8
3	9.8	42.6	75.5	108.3	141.1	173.9	206.7	239.5	272.3	305.1
4	13.1	45.9	78.7	111.5	144.4	177.2	210.0	242.8	275.6	308.4
5	16.4	49.2	82.0	114.8	147.6	180.4	213.3	246.1	278.9	311.7
6	19.7	52.5	85.3	118.1	150.9	183.7	216.5	249.3	282.2	315.0
7	23.0	55.8	88.6	121.4	154.2	187.0	219.8	252.6	285.4	318.2
8	26.2	59.0	91.9	124.7	157.5	190.3	223.1	255.9	288.7	321.5
9	29.5	62.3	95.1	128.0	160.8	193.6	226.4	259.2	292.0	324.8

ENGLISH GALLONS TO LITRES (100 gallons = 454.35 litres)

Gallons	0	10	20	30	40	50	60	70	80	90
0	Litres	45.4	90.9	136.3	181.7	227.2	272.6	318.0	363.5	408.9
1	4.5	50.0	95.4	140.8	186.3	231.7	277.1	322.6	368.0	413.4
2	9.1	54.5	99.9	145.4	190.8	236.3	281.7	327.1	372.6	418.0
3	13.6	59.1	104.5	149.9	185.4	240.8	286.2	331.7	377.1	422.5
4	18.2	60.6	109.0	154.4	199.9	245.3	290.8	336.2	381.6	427.1
5	22.7	68.1	113.6	159.0	204.4	249.9	295.3	340.7	386.2	431.6
6	27.3	72.7	118.1	163.6	209.0	254.4	299.9	345.3	390.7	436.2
7	31.8	77.2	122.7	168.1	213.5	259.0	304.4	349.8	395.3	440.7
8	36.3	81.8	127.2	172.6	218.1	263.5	308.9	354.4	399.8	445.2
9	40.9	86.3	131.8	177.2	222.6	268.1	313.5	358.9	404.4	449.8

LITRES TO ENGLISH GALLONS (100 litres = 22.01 gallons)

Litres	0	10	20	30	40	50	60	70	80	90
0	Gallons	2.20	4.40	6.60	8.80	11.00	13.20	15.41	17.61	19.81
1	0.22	2.42	4.62	6.82	9.02	11.22	13.42	15.63	17.83	20.03
2	0.44	2.64	4.84	7.04	9.24	11.44	13.65	15.85	18.05	20.25
3	0.66	2.86	5.06	7.26	9.46	11.66	13.87	16.07	18.27	20.47
4	0.88	3.08	5.28	7.48	9.68	11.88	14.09	16.29	18.49	20.69
5	1.10	3.30	5.50	7.70	9.90	12.10	14.31	16.51	18.71	20.91
6	1.32	3.52	5.72	7.92	10.12	12.32	14.53	16.73	18.93	21.13
7	1.54	3.74	5.94	8.14	10.34	12.54	14.75	16.95	19.15	21.35
8	1.76	3.96	6.16	8.36	10.56	12.76	14.97	17.17	19.37	21.57
9	1.98	4.18	6.38	8.58	10.78	12.98	15.19	17.39	19.59	21.79

I. THE WITHAM AND THE FOSSDYKE

You cannot fly to Boston, for it possesses no airport although the surrounding countryside is in fact flat enough for there to have been many aerodromes in the past . . . and indeed there were when it was of vital importance to us all to fight off the potential invading hordes of what we called the Hun. (Actually, you can fly to Boston, if you have in mind the New England version in Massachusetts; home of beans, tea-parties, revolutions and cocktails – and home-from-home of the Pilgrim Founding Fathers, and sanctuary of McCarthy-like witch-hunters. However, the Boston you can't fly to is in olde-worlde England; where the Pilgrims started from and where, in their footsteps or, more accurately, in their wakes, we also start from . . . but in a different direction and with entirely different aims and purposes.)

It is probably most inspiring to fly over Boston (Old England, that is) and see The Wash and the Witham from a perspective that throws them into clear and dramatic focus; but it is also equally intriguing to arrive there by road, rail or, as is more appropriate for this volume, by water. Whether you rush to Boston from a hairy crossing of The Wash (looking for the safety of The Haven) or whether you gently cruise there from an idle afternoon on the Witham (intent on braving the Grand Sluice and all that follows on the morrow) will not detract from your appreciation of the unique, enigmatic and quite incorrigible atmosphere, architecture, activities and archetypes that go to make up the experience that is Boston; the beginning and end of Lincolnshire, or should that read, The Fens?

In the good, olden days, before governments started to tamper with the nomenclature of our socio-geographic cultural heritage; before the Vicar of Bray descended into anonymous mediocrity; before the Ridings of Yorkshire were decimalised into ignominy by the cat's-paws of the whited sepulchres of one of Whitehall's worst farces; before all these things had come about, there was the full-blown County of Lincolnshire. This, one of the largest and proudest of the shire counties, also had its ridings; and not the least of the Parts of Lincolnshire (with the greatest of respects to Kesteven and Lindsey) was the Part called Holland. One of its claims to fame was the historic port of Boston; indeed, although the Part known as Holland is now long gone, the port is still revered, and, what is more, is undergoing quite something of a revival under the expert guidance and propulsion of its recently appointed harbour master of substance, one Captain Hulland. What's a vowel between friends? There may be no thought in the minds of the city fathers of emulating their predecessors, the famous Pilgrim Fathers, nor of wreaking havoc in the New England states in revenge for the Boston Tea Party; and while these worthies may not even begin to approach the calibre of their merchant adventurer ancestors,

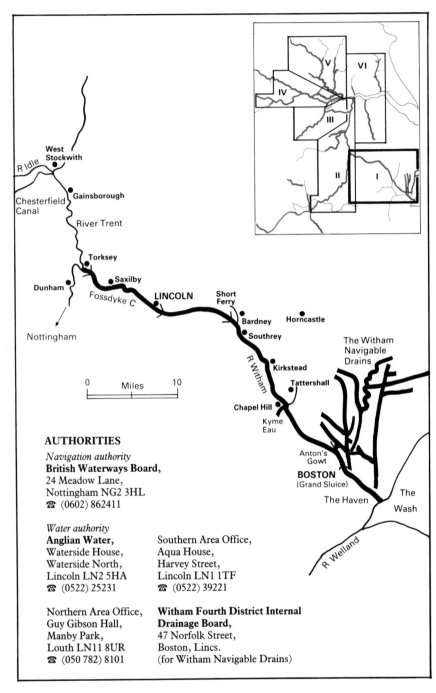

West Stockwith

R Idle

Chesterfield Canal

Gainsborough

River Trent

Torksey

Dunham

Saxilby

Fossdyke C

LINCOLN

Short Ferry

Bardney

Horncastle

Southrey

The Witham Navigable Drains

Nottingham

R Witham

Kirkstead

Tattershall

Chapel Hill

Kyme Eau

Anton's Gowt

BOSTON (Grand Sluice)

The Haven

The Wash

R Welland

0   Miles   10

AUTHORITIES

Navigation authority
British Waterways Board,
24 Meadow Lane,
Nottingham NG2 3HL
☎ (0602) 862411

Water authority
Anglian Water,
Waterside House,
Waterside North,
Lincoln LN2 5HA
☎ (0522) 25231

Southern Area Office,
Aqua House,
Harvey Street,
Lincoln LN1 1TF
☎ (0522) 39221

Northern Area Office,
Guy Gibson Hall,
Manby Park,
Louth LN11 8UR
☎ (050 782) 8101

Witham Fourth District Internal Drainage Board,
47 Norfolk Street,
Boston, Lincs.
(for Witham Navigable Drains)

WITHAM AND FOSSDYKE

Distances
Boston Grand Sluice to Torksey (junction with River Trent) 43 miles (non-tidal).
Boston to The Wash 6 miles (tidal).

Dimensions
Length 75′
Beam 15′
Draught 6′ (but see text)
Air draught 9′ (but see text)

Locks 3

Traffic
Mainly light pleasure craft, but with some larger sea-going vessels on passage to The Wash; BWB craft are also to be encountered, from small tug/tenders to quite large barges.

Remarks
The bridge in Lincoln known as the Glory Hole or High Bridge is the traditional hazard for air draught, but in fact, is not the lowest, nor is it necessarily the most difficult to negotiate. All the bridges in Lincoln demand careful manoeuvring if the craft is anywhere near any of the limits: in particular with a beam of 15′ at the air draught height of 9′. The shallowest stretch is to be found by Branston Island.

OS Maps (1:50 000)
131 Boston & Spalding
122 Skegness
121 Lincoln

Table of distances

	Boston	Anton's Gowt	Langrick	Chapel Hill	Dogdyke	Tattershall	Kirkstead	Southrey	Bardney	Five Mile Bridge	Washingborough	Lincoln	Saxilby	Torksey
Boston		2	4	10	11	12	16	20	23	26	29	31	36	41
Anton's Gowt	2		2	8	9	10	14	18	21	24	27	29	34	39
Langrick	4	2		6	7	8	12	16	19	22	25	27	32	37
Chapel Hill	10	8	6		1	2	6	10	13	16	19	21	26	31
Dogdyke	11	9	7	1		1	5	9	12	15	18	20	25	30
Tattershall	12	10	8	2	1		4	8	11	14	17	19	24	29
Kirkstead	16	14	12	6	5	4		4	7	10	13	15	20	25
Southrey	20	18	16	10	9	8	4		3	6	9	11	16	21
Bardney	23	21	19	13	12	11	7	3		3	6	8	13	18
Five Mile Bridge	26	24	22	16	15	14	10	6	3		3	5	10	15
Washingborough	29	27	25	19	18	17	13	9	6	3		2	7	12
Lincoln	31	29	27	21	20	19	15	11	8	5	2		5	10
Saxilby	36	34	32	26	25	24	20	16	13	10	7	5		5
Torksey	41	39	37	31	30	29	25	21	18	15	12	10	5	

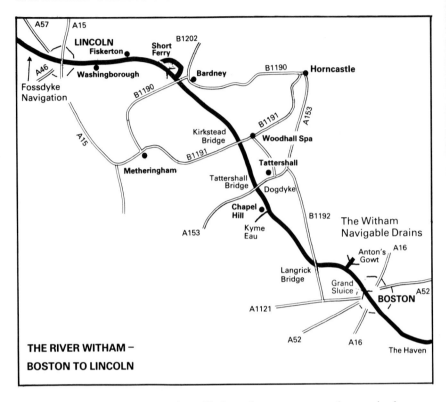

THE RIVER WITHAM –

BOSTON TO LINCOLN

they seem to have every intention of being adventurous merchants – in the general life of the town and port that is, if not, in fact, when it comes to the stretch of river that the observer spies when he looks from the bridge by the Grand Sluice toward the waters of The Wash. The river from the Grand Sluice down to the commercial docks is a disgrace, although still known generally by its more than euphemistic title of The Haven. It may need more than just a little imagination to put the river and its frontage to rights; but it certainly wouldn't cost much in terms of finance, time or even effort; and it is a task that should be undertaken soon for the banks and river bed are all foul for a considerable distance downstream from the Grand Sluice. Even if the town nabobs have little care for the needs of pleasure craft, they should at least respond with enthusiasm to a scheme that would pay for itself over and over again by the monies brought into the presently dead and downtrodden area by committed and well-heeled sightseers. Even the eelers who proliferate along the stretch would welcome such a move, which would make it less likely that they would lose so many nets, tackle and gear. Decent moorings would command a good price, and the riparian neighbours would get nothing but a good deal – in both aesthetics and cash.

Opposite: The Boston Stump.

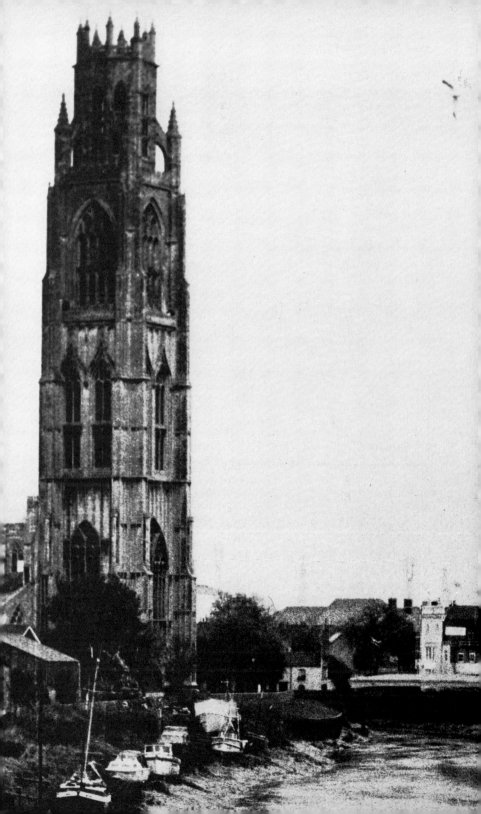

BOSTON LOCK

British Waterways Board
Grand Sluice Lock,
Tattershall Road,
Boston, Lincs.
☎ Boston (0205) 64864
VHF channels: 16 and 74

Restricting dimensions　55' x 26'
Rise and Fall　(tidal)
Mechanised　●
Keeper operated　●
Facilities nearby

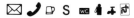

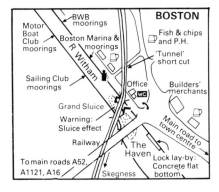

BOSTON

Lincoln 30 miles
The Wash 6 miles

Moorings
British Waterways Board: Lock-keeper Grand
Sluice. Boston Marina (see below).

Marina
Boston Marina, Witham Bank, Boston
☎ (0205) 64420
You will find anything you want here, within
cruising reason, that is. Whether arriving or
departing, Wash or Brayford Pool bound, Mrs
Farmer will tend to your needs and wave you in
or off personally. You can be assured of a real
welcome, patient attention and service well
beyond the calls of duty or commerce. The dog
will also attend your person.

Boatyard
There is no shortage here of people who will
assist maintenance and/or repair. Pre-eminent,
and offering a comprehensive service is the old
established family business of R. Keightley &
Son. They love boats and are to be found at
their yard: Willoughby Road, Boston.
☎ (0205) 63616

Clubs
Approaching Boston from upstream, on what
is known locally as 'the Fresh', on the right
hand bank you will come across the first of the
clubs. This is the hand-powered coterie who
row the stretch in any kind of weather; on the
same side and almost immediately after them
are the powered boats of the Boston Motor Boat
Club; and finally, just before the whirlpools of
the Grand Sluice are the moorings of the
Witham Sailing Club.

Remarks
Boston has all the facilities that any visiting
cruising man can rightfully expect, and a good
many more. Throughout the long straight
approach downstream to Boston and its famous
Stump and Sluice, there is plenty of deep, clear
water. You may see a seal languishing away and
you may get entangled with the lines of some of
the fishermen who seem to be incapable of not
casting immediately in front of any boat that
just happens to be passing by. Near to the
Grand Sluice it is worthwhile looking out for
floating bleach bottles with too much plastic
rope floating from them – since some of the
eelers are not too careful about what they leave
hanging around in the waters, especially when
it is just before or just after the boating season
has started. During the 5 months after
November 1st, it is worth while checking with
Anglian Water at their Boston office about
their plans for lowering the level of the
Witham. ☎ Boston (0205) 65661.

However, as things are, the enormous and enormously unprepossessing construction of the Grand Sluice stands as a suitable symbol for the singularly unbeautiful river that is the Witham below the lock. There has been a sluice at Boston, to protect the Witham from tides and floods, since 1766; and apart from the lock-keeper's standard-issue pill box (from which he controls the doors from a massive array of knobs, switches and lights) and his nearby miniature office, complete with telephone answering service, there is little to convince any passer-by that everything else is not less than two hundred years old. Nevertheless, ancient or otherwise, the Grand Sluice and its associated lock doors is a veritable *watershed* for any visitor or cruising man. Collins dictionary defines as follows: 'dividing line between two adjacent river systems, such as a ridge' or 'an important factor that serves as a dividing line'. Well; the gates and doors are veritably ridges, and there is a clear dividing line between the tidal and non-tidal water of the Witham. There could hardly be a more dramatic difference between the facts and the ambiances of the two connected waters than is to be found in the fresh and in the salt sides of the River Witham. A favourite game of Winnie the Pooh's was called 'Poohsticks'; and it consisted of dropping a stick on one side of a river or stream bridge and then leaning over the other side to watch its journey away into the distance. With or without Poohsticks, it is still a rewarding and revealing pastime to move from one side of the bridge to another (traffic permitting) and contemplate the many contrasts, comparisons and conjectures that the differences will prompt or precipitate: generally speaking, the downstream view is one of rough and tumble waters in a mud and stone ravine; while the upstream consists mainly of not inexpensive craft idling at their mooring places, while their owners dream of waters far away or imbibe in the nearby Witham Tavern. Downstream is all gloom and threat, while upstream is a leafy glade filled with the British Waterways Board's rich promise of a cruising paradise . . . provided your craft in no way exceeds the most pessimistic limitations of the restrictions according to draught (a vessel that draws more than 3′6″ cannot be said to be best suited to the always shallow, often silted and occasionally weeded-up waters of the Witham and Fossdyke and although *Valcon* has made her sometimes erratic and sometimes dead-slow progress from Boston to Torksey on many occasions, her six feet of draught are really far too much to allow a cruise under such circumstances to be called anything but anxious or uncomfortable). However, although there are considerable problems affecting the progress of any boat drawing more than four feet when coming up the tidal Witham early on the tide, there is no parallel of any kind in the waters of the fresh Witham for at least ten miles upstream.

Out of season, the moorings are usually deserted except for the occasional dog, secretly-smoking small boys, equally secretive adulterers, and an amazing old lady who talks to herself, for all to hear, about the world, the flesh and the devil from behind and under a vast conglomeration of cloaks and scarves. Unlike some resorts, Boston has a season that stops and starts with absolute, definite dates; from the first day of November to the last day of April, all mooring is prohibited between the Grand Sluice and any point on the river that may

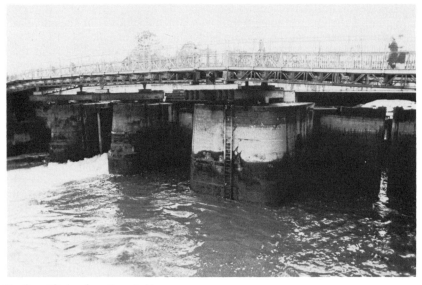

The Grand Sluice: from the salt side.

The Grand Sluice: BBC TV filming *The Grain Run;* inside the lock chamber.

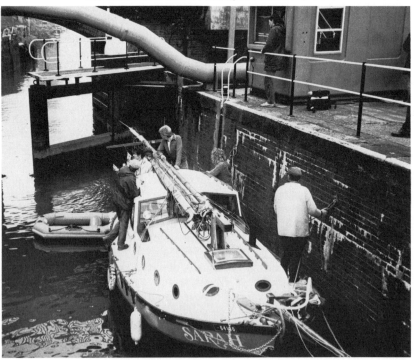

be immediately affected by any speedy sluicing operations that take place to combat flooding or to permit repairs to be carried out to the miles of bank. The sailing and cruising clubs uproot their scaffolding, buoys and finger pontoons; and the more permanent fixtures belonging to Boston Marina and the British Waterways Board become apparent as they are denuded of the craft that have clung to them throughout the summer like so many giant-size limpets – be they *Patella vulgata* or *Ancylus fluviatilis*, one for the salt and one for the fresh.

In season, it is hardly ever quiet, even in the middle of the night, since that favourite occupation, 'messing about in boats', is always much more concerned with the verb and adverb than with the noun, and messing about is, by common consent, unaffected by time, person or place. In addition, there is always someone intent on making tea or coffee, or dispensing alcohol in large or small doses, if not actually to all-comers then at least to all those who are prepared to pay the price of their refreshment by sitting at the feet of some youthful ancient mariner *manqué*, and hearing quite impossible tales of derring-do.

But no matter how strong the lure of the water, the waterside or its seasonal inhabitants, Boston is a place that must be tasted shoresides if it is not to be considerably undervalued. Now, some cruising havens promise the promised land from the water, but on close inspection fail to deliver the goods, in some cases actually disappointing the visitor so intensely that a swift retreat to the water is necessary for survival. (Walton-on-the-Naze is one such case: the approaches are all attractive and filled with eastern coastal promise, but the place itself is so unpleasant (being dirty and noisy) that even stout Cortez would have failed to be silent – albeit while all his men looked at one another with a definitely wild surmise.) But Boston is not of this league. You have only to take your gaze from eye-level to roof to discover visions of architectural glory mainly, it must be said, dominated from almost any viewpoint or angle by the 272′ high tower of St. Botolph's Church, known much better as the famous Boston Stump. There are two market days, Wednesday and Saturday, and while both are good for normal market fare (or even fair or fayre), on Wednesday there are two sites, and the sights to be seen in the open market place near the main post office are almost worth waiting six days to encounter (should you haply arrive on a Thursday) since they range from Aaron's Beard and Aaron's Rod to Zoysia, *Zygophyllaceae* and Zymometers. In addition, there is the thrill of the chase – since all the stallholders welcome any customer who enjoys the cut'n'thrust of barter, bring and buy and auction. Away from the market and the mainstreams of supermarkets and all the usual well-known high street brands and names (for Boston is not to be left behind in commerce though it may seem at times to be more mediaeval than modern) there are back streets and lanes that should not be overlooked, for there you will find the indigenous tradesfolk. In no other market town or harbour have I met so many tradesfolk who are also gentlefolk: always ready to do a deal there and then; equally ready to stand and talk and do no deal at all; more than ready to send you down the road and round the corner to a colleague (who just happens to be a friend or relative) who will be able to oblige you when the first one fails; and nary a one who will do you down or send you up. Boston must surely have its share of thieves, vagabonds and cheats; but I am happy to say that I have never yet had the misfortune to do business with a single one of them.

I am always sorry to leave Boston behind (whether I am going into The Wash or just up the river) and always lay the flattering unction to my soul that it will not be for quite a time that I shall be without a good view of the famous Stump that surveys all around for many a mile. (And for any keen Christian, it is worth noting that you have hardly lost sight of the Stump up the Witham than you are contemplating the massive monument on the hill that is Lincoln's cathedral.)

Once having cast off from the environs of the Grand Sluice, you are likely to encounter sailing, rowing and fishing right up to Anton's Gowt. Sometimes this can be irritating but more often it is pleasing to be able to break up what would otherwise be an unbroken and pretty monotonously straight run to Anton's Gowt. (There is a place on the River Ore in Suffolk that is known as Cuckold's Point and it shares with Anton's Gowt the distinction of being so secret about its derivation that no-one I have asked knows the reason for the odd nomenclature. It so happens that a gowk is a cuckoo, but that is not quite near enough to help, not even when it also means a fool – especially one of the April variety. Any reader who can throw light upon either is asked to do so.) Apart from being oddly named, Anton's Gowt is also the gateway to a really odd set of cruising grounds: the Witham Navigable Drains. Here at least there is no doubt about meaning since it is all straightforward and above board: they are all artificial cuts or old streams and rivulets that have been improved over the years to provide an efficient drainage system for the west and east fens, and they all lie in an area that is to the north of the Witham and to the south of a line drawn from Spilsby to Dogdyke. In years gone by, these Drains were much used for the transport of wood, coal and all sorts of agricultural produce; nowadays they are mainly used for their 'official' function of drainage, and only a little for cruising and fishing. It is indeed some long time since the navigation rights were used in any serious manner. (Although, just like the River Idle, the waterway possesses its enthusiasts who are utterly devoted to ensuring that these rights are not eroded nor fall entirely into disuse.) Only those with really suitable craft should attempt to cruise the area, and then only after proper consultation with the appropriate authorities. At best, the Drains are restricted to craft no more than 60′, and this length will mean there are very few places where it is possible to turn round when meeting an impossible bridge, so it is better to consider an overall length of 30′ with a beam of 11′ (better is 10′) an air draught of 8′ (better is 6′6″) and a water draught of 3′6″ (and this in no way guarantees an unhindered progress). The levels may be dropped from time to time without warning and skippers have been known to be stranded for more than just a short weekend. The Drains themselves are by no means the way to beautiful scenery or grand sights, since the area is generally flat and the Drains are 'guarded' by high banks since most of them are well below the level of the surrounding land. Perhaps the most interesting 'trip', except for those who are never properly satisfied until they have navigated the very last creek and silted arm, is into the middle of Boston. However, once you are in, you are in for good – until you return to Anton's Gowt, for there is no way that the Drains now connect with any other waterway. It is amusing to note that it is still possible to cruise from Boston to New York via Bunkers Hill. The Drains themselves are the proud possessors of some unusual names: Maud Foster, Hobhole, Cowbridge, Bolingbroke, Lush's, Bellwater and Howbridge. There are also many branch lines that are completely without benefit of baptism, although in fact most are known by some name or other to the (very local) locals.

Many people use the lock at Anton's Gowt, or the British Waterways Board's new pilings, just for an overnight stop away from the bright lights of Boston's *dolce vita*. There is little that happens here, for, in spite of the pub, the place is quiet, little visited and almost, but not quite, away from it all. As such, it is just the spot for those who delight in the remote.

ANTON'S GOWT LOCK

The lock is quite remote and there is no lock keeper on duty. However should you require the address it would be
British Waterways Board
Anton's Gowt Lock,
Boston, Lincs.

Restricting dimensions   60' x 16'9"
Rise and Fall   see remarks
Hand operated   ●
Boater operated   ●
Facilities nearby   ⌂ ♪

There is a public house within a few yards of the lock together with a public telephone. Otherwise services are at Boston.

Remarks
Water levels both in the Navigable Drains and on the River Witham vary and so we cannot quote a typical drop in water levels through the lock. However the dimensions in terms of boat size are 60' long x 16'9" wide (BWB). The author recommends a maximum draught of 3'.

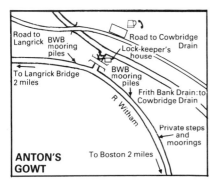

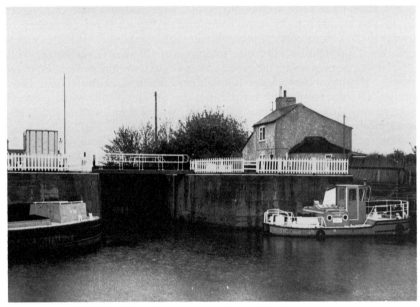

Anton's Gowt: the locked entrance to the Witham Navigable Drains .

Another long, straight stretch goes from Anton's Gowt to the next indication of civilisation: Langrick Bridge. Langrick is just about five miles from Boston and Anton's Gowt is halfway between. With a boat drawing more than a metre, you will find it difficult to moor at the river banks or by the bridge itself; and even with less draught there is no landing stage to give easy access to the facilities that are immediately next to the bridge (general stores, garage and public house with food). The road traffic tends to thunder along and I have never found the spot to be attractive enough for me to put up with the inconvenience of getting ashore. However, it is only an hour's cruise from Boston and therefore quite an attractive proposition for a quiet evening run.

A further hour along the river will bring you to a most intriguing stretch, that to be found between Kyme Eau (locally known as Sleaford Cut) and the old (now disconnected and disused) Horncastle Canal. The first sign of waterborne civilisation comes with the private moorings in Kyme Eau. This waterway used to be known as the Sleaford Navigation and just before the turn of the 18th century (1794 in fact) the 12 miles from the town of Sleaford to the junction with the River Witham were completely navigable. However, ever since 1878 (when the canal was abandoned by Act of Parliament) it has been regressing into decay.

I always think of the three communities of Chapel Hill, Dogdyke and Tattershall as but one settlement divided, like Gaul, into three parts and overlooked (if not overseen or administered) by the last and the largest, Horncastle. The wholly pure indigenes, that is, those locals who have always lived there and

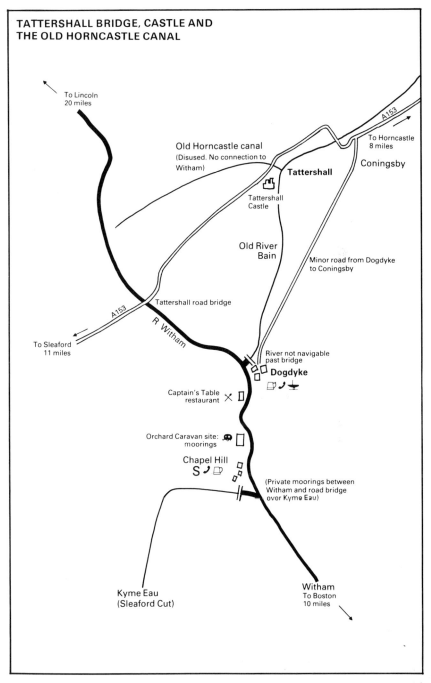

**TATTERSHALL BRIDGE, CASTLE AND
THE OLD HORNCASTLE CANAL**

To Lincoln
20 miles

A153

To Horncastle
8 miles

Old Horncastle canal
(Disused. No connection to
Witham)

Tattershall

Coningsby

Tattershall
Castle

Old River
Bain

Minor road from Dogdyke
to Coningsby

Tattershall road bridge

A153

R Witham

To Sleaford
11 miles

River not navigable
past bridge

Dogdyke

Captain's Table
restaurant

Orchard Caravan site:
moorings

Chapel Hill

(Private moorings between
Witham and road bridge
over Kyme Eau)

Kyme Eau
(Sleaford Cut)

Witham
To Boston
10 miles

whose ancestry goes back into the mists of time and the equally dense mists of the fens, drains, streams and culverts that criss-cross the region, are actually few and far between, but there is a distinctly local quality of character that imbues those who stay long enough to be accepted as 'belonging'; and it is this feeling that is discernible in all the people you are likely to meet while shoresides.

In some parts of Britain it takes years or decades for a 'stranger' to be accepted into the local fold. In some cases, the length is measured in a lifetime, and the individual concerned may even then not be accepted as a qualifier even though he hardly moved out of the village – and finally died there. The extreme north coasts of Devon and Cornwall are such places; but the neighbourhood of Horncastle, Chapel Hill and Dogdyke is no such place: in fact, you may well be welcomed on behalf of the communities as a long lost friend by people who have themselves been there for no more than a few years. Such is the generous-hearted friendliness of the place that you will also be well received by those who can go back generation after generation . . . that is, if you possess the spirit of genuine good neighbourliness yourself and present your person to them accordingly.

CHAPEL HILL AND DOGDYKE

Boston 10 miles
Lincoln 20 miles

Moorings
The well-protected berths and pontoons in Kyme Eau, known locally as Sleaford Cut, are all private, but I have never found the owners to be obsessively territorially minded. In addition, there are stagings at the Orchard Caravan Park, the Captain's Table and the River Bain.

At all of them it is possible for a craft with 6′ draught to get right to the side without too much difficulty although there is a good deal of silt on the Bain side of the river at Dogdyke. There are also plenty of places where a land anchor can be used.

Boatyard
There is an incipient yard at Dogdyke on the old River Bain. In the beginning of 1985, they were only just getting things under way; but now there is a small marina and comprehensive services including such luxuries as showers and tea rooms. ☎ (0526) 42124.

Club
The only club in the area is the one run by Orchard Caravans, and it would take strong competition to get close to them for friendly service. There is 6′ by the berth and you are close to most things that you need, and there is a pleasant short riverside walk to the village.

Facilities

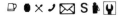

Remarks
With the Crown Inn at Chapel Hill and the Packet Inn at Dogdyke there is good choice for a pint. If you are feeling like eating you can do so there, or in slightly different style at the Captain's Table, where there is also a private mooring for patrons. You will be welcomed with open arms at all three!

However, just one word of warning: these are not folk who take kindly to condescension even in the mildest or slightest degree; and any foolhardy soul who ignores the rules, the facts or the conventions will soon find himself in danger of losing his berth, his facilities and his contacts with the village. In a way, many of them are like Raymond Chandler's heroic private detective, Philip Marlowe: 'a lonely man and his pride is that you will treat him as a proud man or be very sorry you ever saw him.' In brief, you don't need to go to lengths to win them over; but if you even think of relating with them like that you are bound to lose. They will not gain, but you will surely be the poorer. If it is to do no more than meet as many of these quite special local folk as you can, it is well worth a break in your cruising of at least a couple of days; and since there are plenty of facilities around and about there can hardly be a justification for not doing so. For those who like the nether parts of Torksey and prefer a minimal wooden staging or a well planted land anchor to a plastic-coated marina, this couple of miles will take a lot of bettering.

Kyme Eau is the province of Anglian Water and they are issuing all kinds of promises that they will be improving the reach for a few miles in the very near future. As things are, the bridge marks the head of navigation for most people and most purposes (and, in addition, is one of quite a few in the area on which you stand with one foot in one political, parochial patch and one foot in another). Chapel Hill offers a triumvirate to serve you: the grocer (and post master) stocks far more than any boater has any right to ask and seems always to be to hand; the landlord of the local also offers a comprehensive service that is up to the standards of any small hostelry and seems always to hand when really needed, but, out of season, is not against keeping his bar doors barred against intruders while he has thirty-nine winks over the odd lunchtime in the dead of winter; and the keepers of the garden ('orchard' properly means a gar-den-yard: *hortyard* was one of its old spellings from the latin *hortus*, a garden) or the landlords of the caravanserai (an hospitable establishment enclosing a park for covered houses on wheels) will keep or lord you (as is their wont) and make you welcome as befits any honoured guest – even better, they will leave you alone when you are content to be left to your own devices. A triumvirate that can be so prodigal with its talents and services must rate among the best in the land.

The following is what Orchard Caravans say about themselves and the area, and I for one have no disagreement with their remarks:

> The Witham is well known for its coarse fishing and is a growing attraction for boats with access to The Wash, Trent and canal system. Pleasure and match fishing, moorings, winter storage for a limited number of boats or caravans are but only part of the attractions here.
>
> The peace and quiet of the country, wildlife and many places of interest are within easy reach, including Lincoln Cathedral, Boston Stump and mar-ket, Woodhall Spa championship golf course, Spalding Bulb Festival, Skegness, Tattershall Castle and Aero Museum, Dogdyke pumping station to mention but a few.

The toilet blocks have hot and cold water and showers available 24 hours a day during the season. There is a bathroom, drying room, laundry and ironing facilities.

A heated swimming pool is open June to September, plus paddling pool and sand pit with swings for all ages.

A fully stocked site shop with most things the holiday maker requires from bread, milk, frozen and tinned foods, sweets, cigarettes, ice creams, minerals, postcards, some fishing tackle, Calor and Camping Gaz, etc. Ready cooked chickens supplied 24 hours noticed required.

The Long House Club and Bar, full membership or holiday membership (max. 2 weeks) available, is centrally heated and has television and lounge facilities.

Just down the river apiece is Dogdyke itself. Here is another trio: a sophisticated restaurant, The Captain's Table with an excellent private staging, but no really successful means of tying up to it; a traditional pub, the Packet, where you are well received for drinks'n'grub; and the first beginnings of a boatyard/marina/hospice just up the cut of the Old River Bain, where there are already moorings of substance if not aesthetic appeal. All being well, in the future it will be easier to get in to the north bank: at the moment, if your draught is much more than one metre, you will experience great difficulty in approaching the side and will only do so by stirring up the bottom.

In this area, almost everything is 'old': the Old River Bain; the Old Ferry that no longer plies for trade; the Old Horncastle Canal that is now disused and blanked off from the Witham at a point where cattle frequently water; Old Tattershall Castle; and the Old Pumping Station. It is not far from Dogdyke to Tattershall Bridge (about a mile) where the A153 crosses the Witham. The traffic at this point can seem to be thunderous, and it looks pretty hair-raising since there is a sharp bend to be negotiated, and some of the vehicles are exceedingly large. Although the basic facilities of grocery and hostelry are to be found by the bridge, sadly there is no easy access to them: most people think of anchoring a little off the bank and approaching it by dinghy. The bridge arches look, at first appraisal, as if they are going to provide a safe and sheltered mooring, but it is foolhardy in the extreme to try this one. The area is not in as good repair as it might be and the bottom near the piles is more or less all foul. If you are really intent upon mooring around here, the most reasonable way is to run the stem gently on to the bank or on to the shoal mud by the side; put out a stern anchor and two lines from each side, and if you are thinking of staying in such a spot overnight, then a decent riding light over the stern would be a sensible precaution.

No more than half a mile from the bridge on the way to Kirkstead is a most attractive and remote spot where once led off the Horncastle Canal. There is an obvious large 'dent' in the bank where the waterway is now dammed, and this is an excellent place to nudge or nestle your way to the side and settle down in peace and quiet. Not far away across the fields, along the canalside, or along the A153 Sleaford to Coningsby road, there is the small village of Tattershall; and not far away from them is the airfield and a collection of pits and quarries. It is best to ignore these latter (and certainly the airfield and its noisy excesses) and make your quarry the village and remains of the castle built for Ralph Cromwell in the 15th century. Only the keep now remains, but it is in much better repair than many of the other ancient buildings on this route, and the original was an interesting example of brick work with stone used only for some window and door frames.

The Horncastle Canal was built at the turn of the 19th century, but the 10 mile stretch between the Witham and Horncastle only had a short-lived existence, being abandoned in 1885. Remains of the first lock can be seen quite close to the river and some of the lengths are still with water near the town. At one time it served to furnish water to the moat of the castle. There is nowhere in reach for young hopefuls to live it up; the area is one for slow moving souls with a penchant for contemplation.

Moving leisurely along the river to the next port of call occupies about an hour at 3-4 knots and brings nothing in the way of intrigue, mystery, high drama or visual splendour. Birds appear, disappear and reappear regularly along this stretch and in recent years herons have been making something of a comeback, and it is more than likely that you will have a chance to strike up a nodding acquaintance with at least one on this leg. I have always found their scrutiny of passing humanity close to unnerving, and their calculated last-minute departure (apparently so slow but in fact effortlessly, subtly and accurately timed and then efficiently executed) almost disdainful. It is only after they have taken off and landed four or five times still in complete ignorance of the course of the vessel that one realises that their grace and beauty are probably in indirect proportion to their common-sense intelligence. Nevertheless, I would not change one aspect of their behaviour; and certainly have nothing but admiration (and a goodly dose of envy) for their ability to stand absolutely still, on one leg . . . and sometimes with both eyes closed.

Next comes one of my favourite stopping places on the whole of the Witham: Kirkstead Bridge. There is a small community on the east bank (Kirkstead) and an even smaller one on the other (Martin Dales). There is not a lot of life on either side unless you search it out, but the east bank seems to put itself out more to welcome visitors (especially if by boat) than the west – except that if you are a dedicated fisherman you will probably favour them in the opposite order.

Woodhall Spa itself is only just over a mile away (an excellent walk if the weather is clement; and at the right time there are some of the best blackberries in the country for the picking). To get to it you walk through the small riverside community, and here too life goes by at a gentle pace and you will not be pressed by anyone to do (or not to do) anything in a great haste. If you are cruising that way in the middle of winter and need a sack or two of coal to be dropped off you will find the local dealer will come as near as he can to the mooring without thought of a call-out charge or that 'little extra' for the special delivery.

KIRKSTEAD BRIDGE & WOODHALL SPA

Boston 15 miles
Lincoln 15 miles

Moorings

Under the new motorway-type road bridge there is a well found landing spot, but with little water close to the edge. More water but less easy landings are to be found just above and below the bridge. A plank helps overcome all problems. Sound land anchors and a fair bit of rope are needed for the bank-sides close to the water are particularly soggy in places.

There is no marina, boatyard or any other facility of that kind.

There are to be found all the expected facilities of a small village in Woodhall Spa – as well as a few that are absolute bonuses if you have a spare hour or two (or a good few spare notes) to spend in the contemplation of fine or refined works of art.

Much cheaper on the purse (and many think easier on the eye) is the searching 'spire' of stone that is all that is left of the once-famous, once-vast Cistercian monastery of Kirkstead Abbey. The stone and earthworks are visible from the road, and the remains are not always guarded by fierce-looking beasts.

Facilities

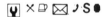

Emergency only: ⚓

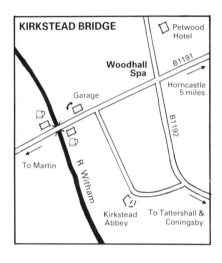

Remarks

There is a garage, telephone, two pubs (one that sells Calor Gas) and a few houses close by. The bridge itself is part of the B1191 Martin to Woodhall Spa road.

Closest to the east bank are the telephone kiosk (usually unvandalised), the Railway Hotel where you will find an individualistic but nevertheless incontrovertible welcome, and Morley's Service Station which does not garishly advertise its presence across the green swards, but which will serve well when you get there.

This less-than-a-hamlet of a place is really well worth stopping overnight (or two) just to relish its peculiar spirit and its few idiosyncracies.

I think Woodhall Spa is a positive dream of a place – except that there is very little about it that you could really call 'positive'. In the main it is vague, and therein lies one of its best attractions. It has not been infected by the contemporary bug of impatient capitalism. No doubt some things have changed (they must have done in the 50 years since I was first taken there as a child) but it feels as if nothing has; and that feeling is all important. You can walk through the village, almost confident that if you were to turn your head fairly sharply you would find yourself being followed by those who lived there centuries ago, just keeping a friendly eye on the old place . . . and a cautious one on you should you be overcome by an attack of modernity and fall into error.

Even if you don't feel like investing days in the pursuit of Woodhall's medicinal mineral springs or tremendous bouts of energy in the pursuit of balls over the springy mineral turf of its famous golf course, do at least allow yourself the indulgence of enough time to ferret out three of the Spa's fascinating features. Almost hidden away in the woods is the Kinema, extremely well named bearing in mind that 'Kinema' is the original spelling of the more common noun cinema, for this 'Kinema in the Woods' has all the airs and graces, if not the actual Graces or even the Muses, of an authentic original cinematograph theatre. After a pleasant tree-lined walk there is the Petwood Hotel, a veritable monument to a life that has almost completely disappeared, but a life that, in its prime, was by no means at one with itself. The *longueurs* that are usually associated with the afternoon tea parties of the rich, the famous and the beautiful were never permitted in the Petwood to gain even a foothold, for there was always the possibility of an onslaught from the forces of the Royal Air Force – and just a chance that one of those revolutionary bombs (for which the hotel has now become deservedly well known) might have been smuggled in by some junior officer suffering from a rush of blood to the brain.

Both the Kinema and the Petwood are, no matter how invested with the lively spirits of times past, nevertheless lifeless monuments and, therefore, in the last resort, no more than things. There is no way that the same can be said of the last member of my trio of memorabilia (and if there was ever a case for 'ferreting out' this must be it, except that it is hardly likely to be needed, so plentiful are the examples of my choice): the squirrel. There are those people who always think of these bright-eyed and bushy-tailed creatures in terms of their immortalisation in the *The Tale of Squirrel Nutkin*, and there are others who prefer to remain cooler about them and refer to them more in dictionary terms; any arboreal sciurine rodent (from *skia* shadow and *oura* tail). These folk then try not to get involved in the arguments about their terrible destructive habits – for there are also those for whom the squirrel is at best a varmint to be raved about – and at anything less than that best a classic vermin to be ruthlessly eliminated. Anyway, whatever your stance, there is plenty to occupy you, and more than enough to see and talk about.

There is neither a lot to see nor to say about Southrey, a small community three miles along the river towards Lincoln. In fact, it seems as if there are two communities,for the ferry that once plied has been defunct for a long time and the bridges are at Kirkstead and Bardney – quite a walk away. So, the two sides are separated by what is at this point the ribbon of the Witham and, to a certain extent, it is a case of east is east and west is west and never the twain shall meet – except for the fact that here it is virtually north and south.

On the north side is to be found Fawlty Towers and the roof-notice warning to airborne navigators to keep their distance (with one of those 'If you can read this, you arc too close' jobs) but a riverside welcome to all waterborne travellers – provided you need little help to moor at the bank, for there is no landing stage and very little water along the whole of that stretch. There used to be a wooden pontoon on the south side giving easy access to the White Horse Inn and caravan park, whose actual address is Dunston Fen, Metheringham, Lincoln, but that got carried away after a travelling troupe departed from it (or failed so to do) with an attack of zeal that would have better been kept for one of their performances. If you are no more than a metre in draught you should have little problem in getting to the bank, and what is more, once you are alongside (and on some occasions well before) you will be greeted by an enthusiastic band of young people (not forgetting the dog!) and can be sure of a helping hand and a warm welcome.

Another three miles up the river comes the lock at Bardney, preceded by the big bend and chimneys that mark the presence of the sugarbeet factory. There is a road bridge near to the actual village of Bardney itself, and I have been advised that it is 'perfectly safe' and also a 'smashing spot to moor'. It looks a tempting spot since there are apparently a number of wooden structures to help the visitor moor and get ashore; but closer inspection shows it all to be a snare and a delusion. The intending caller should firmly resist temptation and move on round the bends and corners and under the heavily girdered bridges that mark the way to the lock at Bardney.

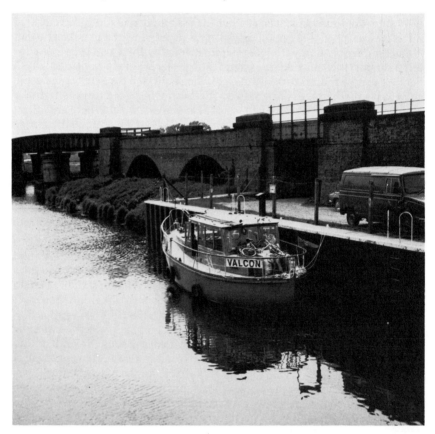

Recent piling has improved access to Bardney Lock; note the conveniently placed water point.

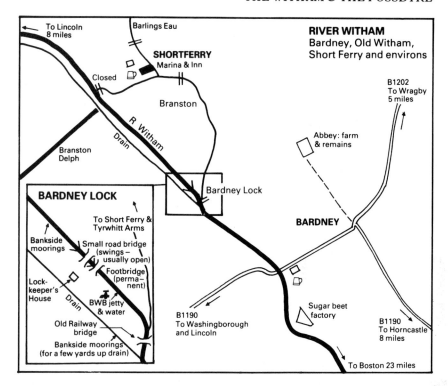

BARDNEY AND SHORTFERRY

Boston 20 miles
Lincoln 10 miles

Moorings

For once, the skipper is faced with a plenitude of acceptable moorings: there are the new piles by the water point which, out of season, are seldom busy enough for you to cause problems by staying there overnight. There is a very quiet patch just up the first drain where there is an open area just in front of the railway arches. There are no facilities or pontoons at this point, but it is very popular especially with the Lincoln cruisers. There are also BWB moorings through the lock on the port hand. They suffer from a lack of water at the bankside; but with a bit of luck, if you need much more than a metre, you should be able to find an hospitable boater who will let you hang on to his outside.

Just before the huge railway bridge at the fork of the river and the dyke there is usually an apology for a notice board advertising the Tyr-

whitt Arms; this hostelry is to be found near the Shortferry Marina by the junction of the old river and Barlings Eau. Access to the marina is restricted on account of both air draught and hull draught: if you are more than 9' in the air and 4' below the water line it is worthwhile contacting the marina manager for his up to date advice – for the water level can change quite considerably (see below). Shortferry Marina, Fiskerton, Nr. Lincoln LN3 4HU. ☎ (0526) 398021.

Facilities

⏚ ● ✕ ⌂ ♪ ⚓ S 📶

Remarks

For skippers who navigate the Boston side of the lock at Bardney, it is worth noting that the water level can fluctuate dramatically enough so that if your air draught is near the limit of the Bailey bridge on the way to Shortferry or of the footbridge at the lock you could find yourself penned or hemmed in after heavy falls. 12" air draught spare space is what is needed for safe comfort. The first mile after the lock on the way to Lincoln carries very little water although in fairness to BWB they have never designated it as a course that has more than five feet and if you are near the six foot mark you will start encountering the bottom, even when at a speed that is no more than floating on the spot as it were. True, the bottom is all soft mud and silt so there is no hazard of submerged rocks; but grits and bits can cause their own kind of devilment in cooling lines and there is always the possibility of jettisoned nastinesses and I have picked up barbed wire, fan belts and on one occasion a mattress from this little stretch. Take care!

BARDNEY LOCK

Restricting dimensions   81'4" x 17'3" x 5'1"
Hand operated   ●
Boater operated   ●
Windlass required   ●
Facilities nearby
At lock   ⚓

In village
not immediately accessible
♪ ⌂ ⌧ **S** ▮

Remarks

No lock-keeper here.

Bardney Lock was at one time manned and since it is having its house refurbished there is every hope that this may come back again but at the time of writing it is as the BWB so charmingly puts it 'boatman operated'. In the lock itself there is a swing bridge on the north wall that is a real pain: it looks inviting to tie up to and to walk on, but in fact offers no decent hold for rope, man, boat nor beast and it is much better to be resolute and turn your back firmly on it and use the much better equipped opposite side.

Having left Bardney road bridge behind and turned left into the final strait before the approach to the lock, you will see the waterway divides ahead of you: one stretch goes directly ahead and the other bends away to starboard – to the north. The one ahead is a drainage dyke that will accompany the Witham all the way to Lincoln; it is the river that takes the turn and having done that immediately turns again to port . . . away from the course of the old river that now leads to Shortferry and does not join the 'canalised' section until a mile or more after the lock. The man-made island is called Branston.

Immediately on the left before the lock is a very new section of piling against which it is a pleasure to tie up: the water is deep; there are plenty of rope holds, hand holds and foot ladders; and there is a close-to water point. The final entry to the lock is guarded by a footbridge which offers an air draught of no more than 12 feet.

I have always found the idea of Bardney more appealing than the actuality of the real thing; nevertheless, I have stayed there many times and have never found it necessary to think any evil thought about the place. Local cruising men have their own specific complaints and at this point the reader is referred to the detailed information for Bardney and Shortferry.

Leaving the lock and the long line of moored vessels behind the next mile has the drain-dyke to one side and the island known as Branston to the other. (Any fans of Branston Pickle are in for a disappointment, for the actual village where they might try to trace its origin and its unique recipe is miles away to the south west, well past Heigh-Ho Heighington and Potterhanworth Booths.) Once past Branston Delph on the left and the chained-off weir and pumping station on the right the danger of finding bottom is more or less over, provided that you keep to a central course.

Five miles from Lincoln comes Five Mile Bridge, a possible stopping off place if you have in mind to visit Fiskerton (known as Fishers' Town when boats used to sail to it on the top of the tide along the Old River Witham when, believe it or not, Torksey was an important port) or the prettily named Cherry Willingham. It is a short (½ mile) walk to the first and about four times as far to the second, but they are both of interest to anyone who cares to dig and delve into the communities that show something of archetypal Lincolnshire at its beleaguered best along what must rank as one of the classic stretches of the Viking Way: long, strong, rough and tough – with the sheep looking just that way in harmony.

A little further along on the opposite bank comes the altogether different community of Washingborough. There is a popular spot where a few 'regulars' are always to be found moored up (access across the drain-dyke is not always easy between Bardney and Lincoln and this is one of the few spots where it is worth crossing it if only 'to get to the other side') but, once again, there is not a lot of water at the side and the boats that are tethered there are by no stretch of the imagination to be called substantial. Nevertheless, Washingborough is not a place to be idly dismissed if you have the few hours it will take to assess the charm and facilities, which are scant on the boating side, but otherwise good, of this dormitory outpost of Lincoln.

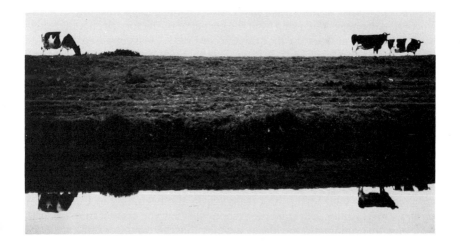

One of the commonest sights in the area: high banks with little life but nature's philosophers.

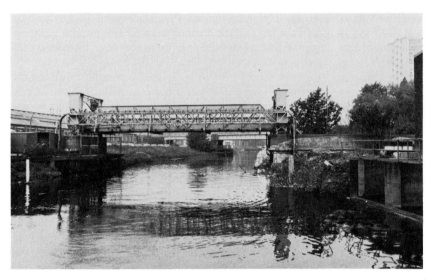

Approaching Lincoln from the south (the Witham): the first bridge; an electrically operated lift bridge – with an operator who is to be summoned from his nearby hideaway.

The first intimation of the presence of Lincoln, apart from the looming spire of the cathedral, which will have been with you for a long time – indeed, you are hardly away from the Stump's supervision from its nearly 300 foot vantage point, than you fall within the aegis of Saint Hugh, are the signs of the power station and factories that go to unglorify this approach. There is always plenty of floating rubbish around here, so it is worthwhile going extra slow. It is also worth it in the hope (often vain) that the keeper of the factory electric lift bridge will see you in time and raise his bridge accordingly. He is supposed to respond to a blast on the whistle, but it is possible that you may have to wait up to a quarter of an hour before someone will allow you to progress through. Once through the bridge, you will reach Stamp End Lock in no time at all, that is, unless you are unlucky enough to find one of the few shoal patches in the last 500 yards before the lock where, presumably, the scouring action of the weir and lock have deposited silt around and about. Here you will be accorded a welcome that may well seem to be low key, but is in fact nothing of the sort. While the keeper is not the man to jump up and down with shouts of glee upon sighting your vessel, you will find that nothing is too much trouble for him and that he is prepared to hang about 'after hours' if you have let him know that you are going to be late. Stamp End really marks the beginning of Lincoln City proper and it is quite clear from the exceptional view you get of it from the lock, what it is that dominates the place. It is possible that you may think there are two dominating institutions hereabouts, for the contemporary architecture of the AWA headquarters does certainly vie with the eight-hundred–year-old cathedral.

STAMP END LOCK

British Waterways Board
Stamp End Lock,
Stamp End,
Lincoln
☎ Lincoln (0522) 25749

Restricting dimensions   81′3″ x 17′3″ x 5′0″
Mechanised   ●
Keeper operated   ●
Facilities nearby

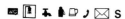 S

Remarks
Hours of operation:
Monday 0800-1730
Tuesday-Friday 0700-1730
Saturday 0700-1200
Boaters are requested to book passage through this lock at least one hour before the level of the tide on which they wish to proceed through the lock. This will allow for the lock-keeper to programme locking and avoid unnecessary delay and inconvenience. Ansaphone facilities are available in the absence of the lock-keeper.

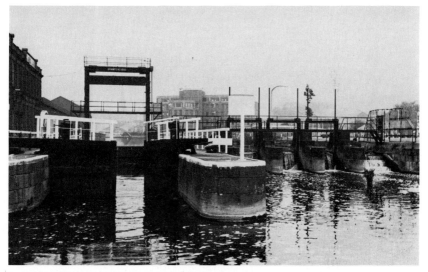

Stamp End Lock and Weir with Anglian Water Offices in the background .

The lock itself is of the guillotine type, and not even the best offices of the keeper can prevent your vessel from being assaulted (in the usual way from a guillotine action) and you would be wise to make sure you have some stout ropes of the appropriate length immediately to hand. The keeper's office is just across the road. There are plenty of places to tie up while waiting – but no facilities in the immediate area, although the shopping centre is not far away.

Next comes a series of pipe, road and foot bridges, including the well known Glory Hole or High Bridge (see the detailed information for Lincoln), and a mile or so of urban waterway that is a great joy and an aesthetic pleasure to look at. The planners have done a good job here; and it's pretty obvious why it is so popular with boaters, tourists, Lincolnians and their swans. In addition it gives easy access to the ancient and modern shopping centres and markets. The only hazard to watch for is that of falling objects, dropped by ladies and gentle-

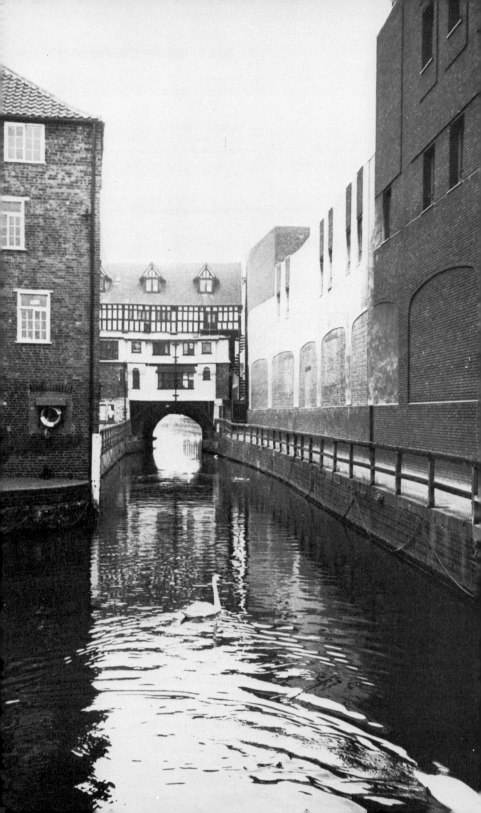

men of uncertain origin, macabre make-up, bizarre hair-style, no fixed abode and an undoubted grudge against the rest of humanity, especially any that happens to pass under the bridge in boats when they may be holding one of their regular sabbats, a ritual part of which is to lean over the parapet and drop on to those beneath any missile that comes to hand, expectorating the while. Sadly, the punk and funk of this world tend to be the junk, the rockers the mockers, the mods the sods and (irony upon irony) the rest the best. However, Lincoln's High Bridge is not the place, neither are its occupants the candidates for any such argument; after all, 'Where ignorance is bliss, 'tis folly to be wise.' And, moreover, 'He who sits beneath a knave should be swift to listen and slow to look up.'

Once through the Glory Hole, there is no more than a modern road bridge to stand between you and the great acreage of Brayford Pool; home of hundreds of cruising enthusiasts (or, if not exactly cruising then certainly boating, for the Pool is a local headquarters for messing about in boats) from far and near.

The Brayford Trustees are to be congratulated on their efforts and their results although there is still much to be dredged on some sides and by the pretty floodlit island. For deeper draught boats, the best moorings are to be found by the harbour master's office (see plan of Pool) and under no circumstances should they venture near the island – although the bottom is clean and free from everything more hazardous than mud.

Life abounds on and around the Pool, and Lincoln has all the facilities that can be asked of a county town. It also possesses enough history and heritage to keep any interested crew shoresides for the best part of a week. I have four favourite shopping stations: two of them are fairly predictable, Sainsbury's (because it is comprehensive in its range and only yards away from the Pool); and the market in the centre of the town (and while some of the stalls show signs that their holders have given in to some of the less pleasing aspects of modernity, there are enough of the traditional kind to make a special journey really worthwhile). The other two are more unusual: Mazurska's, a delicatessen that is also fairly close to the Pool (near the post office) with a proprietor who, if he doesn't have what you want to hand, will take enormous pride and pleasure in obtaining it for you without fuss but with efficiency. The fourth candidate is the (now perhaps nationally known) Whisky Shop. It is to be found in Bailgate, right up the hill near the cathedral. It is something of a long haul from the Pool, but the haul is justified for the joy of discussing with discriminating purveyors of wines and spirits, whiskies and all kinds of spirituous liquors, their virtues, merits, pros and pros (for there really is no contra about any of the liquids, juices or saps that grace their shelves and there is certainly nothing contra to be uttered concerning their *Cointreau*). Their array of single malts (in all kinds of sizes to suit all kinds of pockets, literally and metaphorically) is enough by itself to send a connoisseur into a transport of delight.

The Glory Hole (or High Bridge) seen from the Brayford Pool approach.

LINCOLN

Boston 30 miles
Torksey 10 miles

Moorings

A wide variety: there are clubs, there is the Lincoln Marina, and there are those directly run by the Brayford Trustees, through their harbour master. His office tower is obvious on the north east side. There are all domestic facilities nearby. Fees are not inexpensive, but the berthing is good value for money.

The Harbourmaster,
Brayford Trustees,
Brayford, Pool
☎ Lincoln (0522) 21452

Marina

The Lincoln Marina: Brayford Pool. ☎ (0522) 26896. All facilities except petrol.

Boatyard

There is no boatyard as such, but between Lincoln Marina and C. W. Green (Perkins main agent) as well as the light engineering and electrical businesses around and about, plus the many DIY shops nearby, you should be able to get all the help you might need.

Club

There are many and various clubs in Brayford Pool; but no club could offer you a warmer welcome than that given by the Lincoln Boat Club whose premises are opposite the marina and near the disco on the barge (Bunny's!) and their club night is Fridays, from about 2000.

Facilities

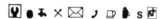

Remarks

There are all the domestic facilities you could ask for; and, on the specific boating side, there is little that is lacking and someone will soon sort you out, even if what you want is not to hand.

Back at the Pool, there is a well-stocked chandlery at Lincoln Marina (known to many as James Kendall Ltd, and directed by Doris Farmer from the

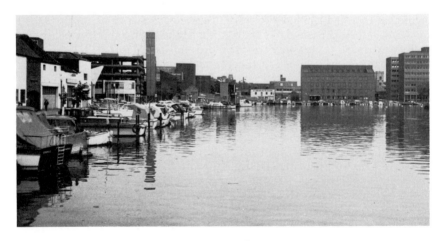

Brayford Pool, with the harbour master's office on the left towards the end; once close to it, you perceive the tower power of Sainsbury's.

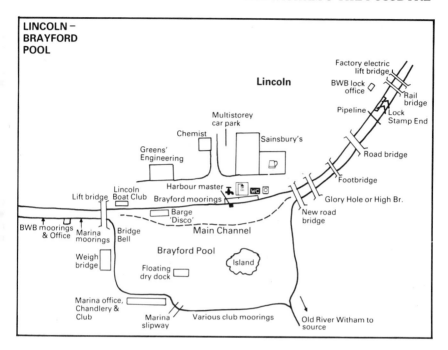

Boston operation) where they also have a clubhouse that is open every weekend. The staff at the marina will do their very best to sort you out no matter how strange your request may appear to be, however, they will do it in their own inimitable manner, for they are all persons of character; personable, characterful, idiosyncratic and with a special kind of home-grown charisma that for all its native origin tends to thrive only on exotic plants.

Also alongside the Pool is the practice of Perkins wizardry that is executed in the name of C. W. Green. Carl (the present day family boss man) is not only an officer of the Brayford Trust but also a keen boating enthusiast himself, aided by his Morse lieutenant who, if anything, is even keener, and one way or another they are likely to be able to help keep you on your watery way if you should need their expertise.

On the way out of the Brayford Pool on the way to Torksey there is a bridge at the end of the Pool. In order to call the keeper you need a BWB Yale key (as for their water and sanitary station points) to unlock the bell. You will often find that he is awaiting you, having been on unofficial lookout; but even if he isn't, he will respond speedily to your signal. The bridge is permanently raised each evening at 1800 until 0600 and for the weekends from Friday 1800 to Monday 0600. After the bridge comes a long line of moorings, the first administered by Lincoln Marina and the next by BWB whose offices are on this stretch. You will find a variety of craft in a variety of states and the moorings seem to go on for a very long time. On the opposite bank is to be observed Lincoln racecourse and its accompanying golf course.

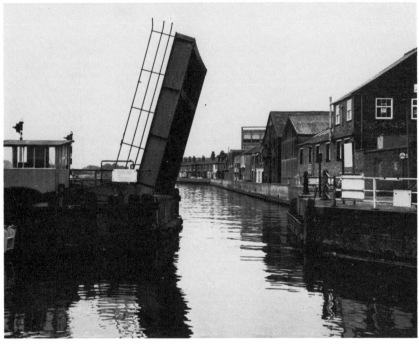

The notice gives instructions about summoning the operator of this bridge which is at the north exit from Brayford Pool – giving on to the Fossdyke.

Not long after, and on the same north side, lies the Pye Wipe Inn. At the time of writing it is still well and truly isolated, with the best approach being by river; but there are major roadworks in the area and soon the place will be humming with a clientele that never before knew that it was there. The external architecture of the place leaves a lot to be desired, but that is well and truly compensated for once you are inside, both appearance and atmosphere being in the best tradition of pub bonhomie. As for that wretched eponymous bird! There are those, so incensed by not being able to get a definitive answer, who steadfastly maintain that it is related to the pye or pie-dog: an ownerless, wild mongrel in Asia; and is also connected with that strange oath, 'By cock'n'pie', although there are, of course, those who claim that all that is no more than a cock'n'bull story. It has actually been whispered to me that the bird is a common lapwing and its name is derived, onomatopoeically, from the sound of its call; and those who make the claim justify it by referring to a classic from the world of literature *Dick of the Fen* who is said to be able to tell better than anyone 'where more piewipes' eggs are'. Anyway, it's good for a lark if nothing else; and if you come up with something earthshattering in terms of research you may be well rewarded by Rod and Nell for when Shakespeare uses the oath, he does so as follows: 'By cock and pie, sir, you shall not away tonight.' (*Henry IV Part II*)

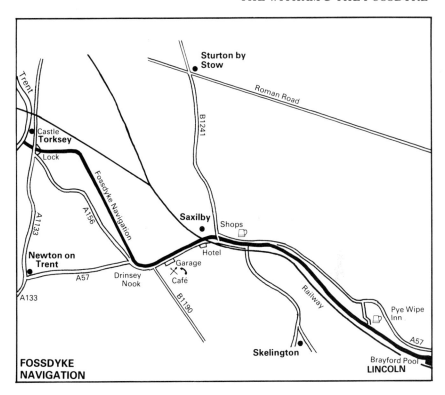

From the Pye Wipe to Saxilby is about four miles and most of the route is fairly low-key in most ways. There are factories on the left bank just before Saxilby and it is not unusual to find working tugs and other craft lurking in the vicinity. (If you draw the maximum for the waterway, you will occasionally need to stand your ground, or water, as the case may be, for some of the working skippers do not readily accept that they have just as much an obligation to make way for craft that are 'constrained by draught' as anyone else. Delicate use of the ship's whistle can be called for.)

Saxilby is a pleasant village with a main street that runs with the canal for a good distance. Within walking distance there are all the facilities you need except for major repairs. Even then, they are a bright lot hereabouts and there is a good chance that someone will be able to improvise and get you on the way again. Within earshot there are two fish and chip shops and three hairdressers. There are also two public houses facing the waterway: one is the Ship Inn, where you will get the kind of welcome that is usually reserved for prodigal sons; you will be offered first-rate beer at decent prices; and you will be given the kind of service that goes well beyond the call of duty or the responsibilities of the Licensing Acts. It is a real joy to patronise the place. The other inn is the Sun.

In the same waterfront stretch is a tucked away agricultural engineers with a splendid D.I.Y. array and a small general stores in the best tradition of corner shops, although it is on the straight. On the other side of the water (with some of the aspects of the other side of the tracks) there is an hotel-type establishment with access from both road and canal.

There are plenty of places to moor along the High Street (with decent fixtures too!) and it is easy to get ashore. There are pipe bridges and rail and road bridges; B.R.'s Inter City 125s tend to make the railway bridge an unpopular spot to tie up, and on occasion the others can be a bit of a hazard because of the presence of dangling adolescents who seem to use them as public service adventure training grounds.

All in all, Saxilby is an intriguing experience, and well worth a stopover be it during the day or night.

Between the village and Drinsey Nook, on the left-hand bank and across the main road, is a garage and upmarket travellers' 'caff'. There is no mooring facility other than the grassy bank – and that can be covered in the season by fishermen and their tackle. Indeed, the next mile or so by Drinsey Nook and after is one of the most piscivorously populated stretches that I have come across on any river or canal; presumably because the access from the main road, where meet the A57(T), the A156 and the B1190, is so good, and there are plenty of facilities nearby. Not all of the fishermen are unco-operative, but conditions can get unfavourable to passing craft.

After Drinsey Nook, there is little in the way of variety until you reach Torksey. Most of the canal is a long straight stretch, and unless you watch from the top of the wheelhouse you will see little of the passing countryside; it is the classic Lincolnshire design, straight and flat with high banks that are also straight and flat. The consolation comes with the wildlife; if you are there when it is not the height of the season and steam along gently and quietly, you will be rewarded by birds a'plenty and water rats in profusion.

Torksey itself is preceded by moorings on each bank, masses of them, and their very presence indicates the popularity of the place. The first sign of shoresides life comes with the Wheelhouse Restaurant. It is a place that I remember well and with some warmth since the proprietor came to my rescue, some few years ago. It was one winter and Anthea and I had been cruising non-stop for nine months in continuous foul weather; and here we were at Torksey at the beginning of a December that had already marked itself for the record books for being wet, cold and windy. On board *Valcon*, we were short of fuel and decent food, and, of course, it was Sunday. Learning of our plight, the lock-keeper suggested that we should knock on the man's door and 'See what happens; you never know, you might be in luck. He's a little on the unpredictable side, but has a heart of gold!' Herbert (for he had not then given up the post to Sid who came after) prophesied better than he knew, for the owner of the Wheelhouse was so overcome by pity for our pathetic sight and plight (it was pouring down and the approach to the restaurant along the bank was a slow plod in the clinging mud) that he actually invited us to join him for a specially prepared feast of good old roast beef and Yorkshire pudding. Long may that particular wheel keep turning.

Then come more wheels as the lock heaves into sight. Here you will be greeted by the keeper, Sidney Rotherham. He is a gentleman, and expects all boat folk to be gentlefolk too; and if that is your inclination, you will find that your stay or passage will be a gentle and pleasurable affair. He is a man of a good many wise saws (quite a few of them original and well worth listening to without interruption) and will go out of his way to guide you not only in and out of the lock (and up and down the Trent's sometimes baffling timetables) but also through that part of life that is, and is symbolised by, Torksey.

I must confess to having a soft spot for Torksey, and for the Witham and Fossdyke generally. All along the 40 miles to Boston there is peace and quiet more or less everywhere you choose to cruise, tie up a line or drop a hook; there are the three exceptional places to stay and explore (Torksey, Lincoln and Boston); and at the west exit there is the challenge or relaxation of the River Trent (dependent upon whether you turn left or right out of Torksey Cut) while at the east there is the ever-changing phenomenon of The Wash. All in all, it must rate as one of the most attractive yet unappreciated, and certainly under-praised, waterways of the UK.

With regard to the Fossdyke Navigation itself, it is by no means a lengthy affair; nor will it win any prizes for being the biggest, the broadest or the most beautiful since it is, in fact, actually ugly in stretches, and cannot claim more than 12 miles at the optimistic count. However, it does possess one important claim to fame: it is the oldest artificial navigation in Britain still to be in use and perhaps the very oldest anyway. It dates from the time of the Emperor Hadrian (about AD 120) who, apparently, had enough spare hours and manpower to be able to dig the Fossdyke and also build his wall. The Romans also made the Witham navigable to Lincoln, and the Fossdyke was cut in order to connect up with it and provide a through waterway from The Wash to the garrisons at York.

The Romans made much use of the link with the Trent and the Humber; and in later years it was also used by the Danes during their invasion and after, and later still by the Normans to carry stone for the cathedral at Lincoln. Torksey is quite different from the other locks lower down the Trent (namely West Stockwith and Keadby) and also the wharfs at Gainsborough, since it is possible to use the entrance to the cut and to find a secure unthreatened berth at almost any state of the tide.

Torksey is the proud possessor of all kinds of intriguing people and places. Undoubtedly the most noticeable (especially from the tideway) is the castle, sadly now little more than a tumble-all-a'crumble and not at all safe to tilt at. Its façade is quite splendid though, and dramatically scans the river from its vacant windows; a river that flows almost to its feet and in times past must have subjected the inhabitants to more than one trial by water.

Close to the old castle is a new bungalow where lives a certain Miss Wickens (of uncertain age but by no means uncertain spirit, certainly not!). The name

TORKSEY

Boston 40 miles
Cromwell Lock 16 miles
Trent Falls 37 miles

Moorings

There is a staging in the Cut where craft of up to 6' draught can lie afloat at all stages of the tide (the part nearest the road bridge is the shallowest). Through the lock there are plenty of places, but there is great competition for the spot is popular. Take the advice of the lock-keeper.

Club

Torksey is a great favourite with cruising clubs.

Facilities

Repairs, diesel and petrol can be obtained but with difficulty.

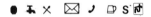

Remarks

Access through the lock to the Fossdyke Canal can be a tricky affair if your craft has a draught of more than 3'; and under such circumstances it is wisest to check with the lock-keeper about the amount of water that he actually is likely to expect at any one tide. Sometimes, when there are neap tides and there has been something of a drought, it is possible to have as little as three feet of water only over the sill. Generally speaking, craft of up to six feet can expect to get in without trouble at high water.

When leaving the cut it is advisable to keep the entrance open until well out into the river as there are silt and mud spits on each side. The lock-keeper will (if requested) check the traffic on the river over VHF; skippers can do the same for themselves if they wish. Once on the river it is wise to monitor the traffic of commercial as well as pleasure craft. The regular channel is VHF 12.

TORKSEY LOCK

British Waterways Board
Torksey Lock,
Torksey,
Lincoln
☎ Torksey (042771) 202
VHF channels: 16 and 74

Restricting dimensions
81'5" x 16'6" x 6'10" (varies)
Torksey to Lincoln 75'0" x 15'3" x 5'
Lincoln to Boston 75' x 15'3" x 4'6"
Rise and Fall (tidal)
Keeper operated •
Facilities nearby

Remarks

Special locking arrangements apply at all times because of tidal conditions. Boaters should contact the lock-keeper direct to programme locking and avoid unnecessary delay and inconvenience.

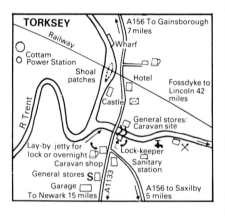

of her abode is *Harmony*, completely apposite for one who will greet your requests to 'view' the castle with olde-worlde courtesy. If your person appeals to her, she may well take you into her confidence and regale you with tales of her unique 'polled' herd, and of her intimate friendships and close encounters over the years with her favourite bulls, who used to graze in the castle grounds. She may also try to enrol your support for a number of ecological causes or conservationist campaigns. In the end, it will make little or no difference; she is likely to enthral you.

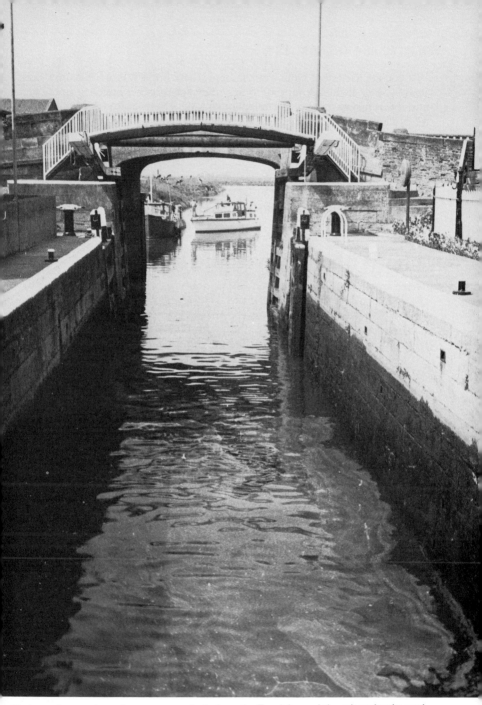

Torksey: the moorings; the entrance to the lock on the Fossdyke; and the exit under the road bridge into the tidal waters of the River Trent. The excellent staging facility can be seen just through the bridge on the left.

If you are in need of liquid refreshment, there is the White Swan only yards away where, at the appropriate times, they specialise in huge log fires. This hostelry is just past the public telephone kiosk. There is also the Hume Arms; the Nicholson Ordnance Survey Guide claims that it is 300 yards away from the junction of the Fossdyke and the Trent while the licensee claims that it is no more than 400. It is in fact half a mile, but still worth the walk for the food and the atmosphere.

So, from the tidal waters of The Wash to the tidal rushes of the Trent: 40 miles of a waterway that seldom gives offence and provides more intriguing stopping off places to the mile than almost any other stretch of cruising waters that I know.

The Witham Navigable Drains

There are those boating folk who will no doubt feel that these 'waterways' are entitled to a full chapter on their own. However, it can only be those whose cruising is never complete unless they have explored (at length and in depth but more often shallowly) every single rod, pole or perch, fathom by careful half-fathom and often are not satisfied until they have found the source, thanks to the use of a skimming inflatable. This guide, however, is for the exoterically (if not indeed vulgar) minded, and not those in search of the last thing in exotica or the esoteric which, in their way, are exactly what the navigable drains are.

The name Witham Navigable Drains is the optimistic title given to those drains that occupy an area north of the River Witham and south of a line from Spilsby to Dogdyke. They are all, first and foremost, functional; being artificial cuts or old streams or courses improved by man, exclusively for the purpose of draining the east and west Fens. Over the years, it became clear to the parsimonious indigents that there was a form of transport going to waste, and the drains were thenceforth pressed into service to carry craft loaded with agricultural produce, wood and coal. Even as recently as 1983 I was cornered by a frugal boating enthusiast who informed me, complete with all the tedious exactitudes that can be marshalled only by a recent and amateur enthusiast, that it was still possible, using only the natural tides and flow, to carry goods completely free of charge from York to The Wash. He hadn't got his licences or dues properly worked out, but his assessment of the principle was sound, falling down only when one asked precisely how long such an expedition would take and how reliable would be any timetable based on such carriage. Nowadays, it is only the drainage factor that is of significant importance although pleasure craft and fishing boats still use the Drains fairly consistently, and are very jealous in the way they exercise their navigational rights, if for no other reason than to remind the authorities (whoever they may be, and that is by no means certain) that there is a common right of navigation to be protected.

On the whole, it is best to take as much local advice as you can get, for the levels can be unpredictable and skippers have been known to be isolated in the

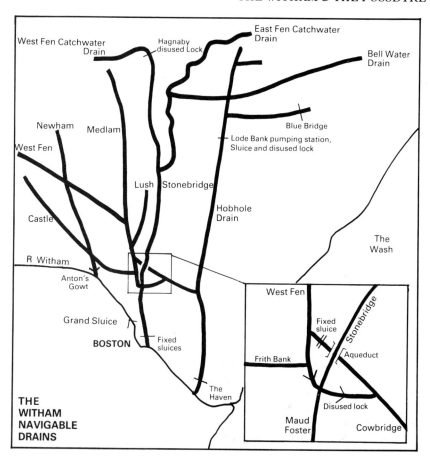

THE WITHAM NAVIGABLE DRAINS

COWBRIDGE LOCK

West Fen Drain (Witham Navigable Drains)

Witham Fourth District Internal Drainage
Board,
47 Norfolk Street,
Boston, Lincs.
(Contact: The Engineer)

Restricting dimensions   71' x 11'6"
Rise and Fall   Up to 3'0"
Hand operated   ●
Boater operated   ●
Facilities nearby

Remarks
No moorings, marina or club. There is a
boatyard: Keightley & Son, 156 Willoughby
Road, Boston. The boatyard is about 1 km
south of the lock on the Maud Foster Drain.
Telephone and pub are at Anton's Gowt, near
Cowbridge and also near the lock. Other
facilities are to be found in Boston, which is 2
miles south of the lock – by road or by Maud
Foster Drain. The key and winding handle to
the vertical lift door is held at Keightley's
Boatyard; and they make a charge if they are
asked to operate the doors.

Drains for a very long time, thanks to an unexpected change in the depth of water affecting his hull draught or his air draught – and it is no joke to be caught above one of the small bridges in the middle of nowhere. However, the Drains do provide some intriguing lengths of navigation for those with craft suited to the adventure. Maximum dimensions, for those with no wish to experiment, are: length 30'; draught 3'; beam 9'; air draught 6'6".

The interested reader is referred to L. A. Edwards' *Inland Waterways of Great Britain.*

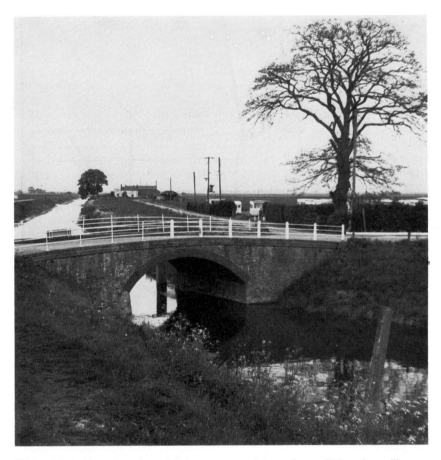

Witham Navigable Drains, where all is always serene and almost always still, but where still waters by no means always run deep.

II. THE RIVER TRENT

Let us not make any bones about it at all: the River Trent is a great waterway. From Derwent Mouth, or thereabouts, it runs for nearly 100 miles to Trent Falls where it joins the Yorkshire Ouse to form the mighty Humber, a river that drains one fifth of England and can dismiss a pleasure cruiser with nary an effort.

The Trent is a very old waterway; dug-out canoes dating from 1000 BC have been found at Nottingham, and the river was constantly exploited by the Romans and the Danes. It was not until 200 years ago, however, that the navigation was knocked into anything like its usable, present shape; and, bearing in mind how little it is now trafficked commercially, it seems difficult to believe that the largest and most recent lock was built at Newark no more than 30 years ago.

Of its nominal 100 miles, 50 are tidal from Cromwell Lock down river to Trent Falls (or Trent End, according to taste); and 30 more will take you up river from Cromwell to Nottingham and its symbol of all that is chauvinistic, namely Trent Bridge. The nearby Meadow Lane Lock takes vessels of suitable draught through to another kind of cruising altogether, but this volume is only concerned with the stretch from Nottingham to the junction with the Yorkshire Ouse; and there can be no greater contrast than between the calm, pond-like waters that run by the city's council offices, British Waterways Board headquarters, the river police office and moorings, Trent Bridge cricket ground, Nottingham Forest football ground and a veritable plethora of water-orientated (if not water-dedicated) clubhouses, and the much more troubled waters of Trent Falls where floods rush in and ebbs tend to slug their muddy ways seawards through a bleak countryside that is only occasionally alleviated by a glimpse of an attractive cottage or the snatched view of an appealing vista. However, before I get completely carried away with the lilies and languors of virtue and the raptures and roses of vice that I constantly associate with the Trent at its best and its worst, let me hasten to add that the River Medway, albeit in an entirely different way, must be a serious contender for the title of Supreme River of Contrasts and Comparisons.

Trent Falls may be approached from the Ouse, the Humber or from upstream; and here we are concerned with the seventy miles that go to make up the cruising ground from Nottingham to this junction, and we shall take it, as they say, 'from the bottom' . . . but first, how did we get here in the first place? In this chapter we are concerned with arrivals from the Ouse or from the Ancholme or the Hull via the Humber; and the questions of what time to leave Hull, South Ferriby, Goole, or any of the other points of call on the tidal Ouse in order to catch a flood tide up the Trent (and it must make sense to try to do that on every trip) are so related to draught and speed of craft as well as neap or spring tides that it requires some special study to get it right every time.

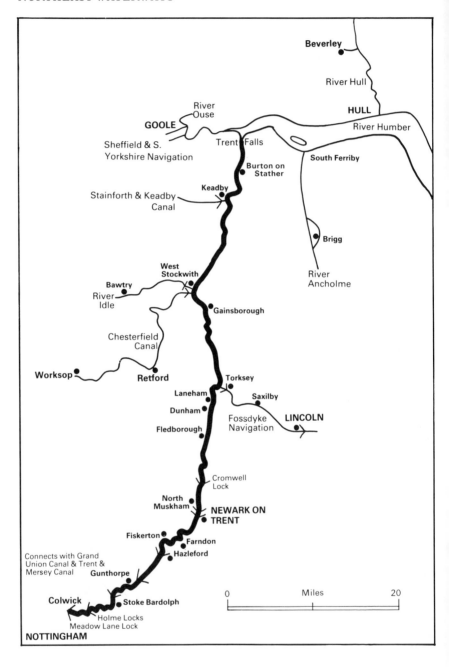

TABLES OF DISTANCES
River Trent

	Trent Falls	Keadby	West Stockwith	Gainsborough	Torksey	Cromwell Lock	Newark-on-Trent	Farndon	Fiskerton	Gunthorpe	Colwick	Nottingham: Meadow Lane
Trent Falls		10	22	27	37	53	58	60	63	70	78	80
Keadby	10		12	17	27	43	48	50	53	60	68	70
West Stockwith	22	12		5	15	31	36	38	41	48	56	58
Gainsborough	27	17	5		10	26	31	33	36	43	51	53
Torksey	37	27	15	10		16	21	23	26	33	41	43
Cromwell Lock	53	43	31	26	16		5	7	10	17	25	27
Newark-on-Trent	58	48	36	31	21	5		2	5	12	20	22
Farndon	60	50	38	33	23	7	2		3	10	18	20
Fiskerton	63	53	41	36	26	10	5	3		7	15	17
Gunthorpe	70	60	48	43	33	17	12	10	7		8	10
Colwick	78	68	56	51	41	25	20	18	15	8		2
Nottingham: Meadow Lane	80	70	58	53	43	27	22	20	17	10	2	

Navigation authority
British Waterways Board,
24 Meadow Lane,
Nottingham NG2 3HL
☎ (0602) 862411

This is the licensing authority for the river between Shardlow and Gainsborough.

Associated British Ports (Hull),
Kingston House Tower,
Bond Street,
Hull HU1 3ER
☎ (0482) 27171

This is the navigation authority up to the South side of the Stone Bridge in Gainsborough. No licence is required.

Water authority
Severn-Trent Water Authority,
Lower Trent Division,
Mapperley Hall,
Lucknow Avenue,
Nottingham NG3 5BN
☎ (0602) 608161

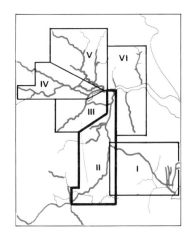

RIVER TRENT

Distances
Trent Falls to Nottingham 80 miles
Trent Falls to Cromwell Lock 50 miles (tidal)
Cromwell Lock to Nottingham 30 miles (non-tidal)

Dimensions
Tidal
  Length unlimited
  Beam unlimited
  Draught up to 10'
  Air draught Keadby Road/Rail Bridge:
      16'9" at MHWS (Rise 15')
      Gainsborough Stone Bridge:
      9' at MHWS (Rise 10')
Non-tidal
  Length 120' (if max. beam)
  Beam 17' (if max. length)
  Draught 6' (but see text)
  Air draught 13'

Locks 8 (including Meadow Lane, Nottingham)

Traffic
Large coasters up to Keadby; smaller coasters up to Gainsborough; and substantial barges up to Cromwell. Pleasure craft from dinghies to sea-going yachts of a substantial LOA. Upstream of Cromwell, mainly pleasure.

Remarks
There is a world of difference between the locked section and the tidal stretches, especially those below Torksey. The use of the Trent Boating Association charts and/or pilot or friendly skipper who knows the waters well, and possesses real local knowledge, must be strongly urged. Any craft navigating the tidal section much be equipped as if for coastal cruising.

O.S. Maps 1:50 000
112 Scunthorpe
120 Mansfield & The Dukeries
129 Nottingham & Loughborough

Charts
These are published by ABP Hull (see above) and cover two areas:
  Spurn to Barton Haven
  Barton Haven to Burton Stather
They are essential for cruising in the vicinity of Trent Falls.

British Waterways Board navigation notes for users of the River Trent between Nottingham and Gainsborough

Weirs
Usually a lock is accompanied by a weir. These weirs are dangerous and should not be approached, particularly under flood conditions. They present a greater hazard when travelling downstream. The following advice is given as though you are approaching the lock heading downstream:

a. Each lock is equipped with traffic lights either side of the entrance – head for these and pass between them.
b. Take note of any signs on the banks telling you to keep left/keep right and then move to that side of the river.
c. On each lock bullnose is a sign telling you to keep left/keep right and this may be accompanied by a directional arrow – keep to the left or right of that sign or move across in the direction of the arrow.
d. The weir approaches may be buoyed or marked at a limited number of locations, i.e. Cromwell Weir. Red buoys or posts with a cylindrical cap – keep to the left of these when travelling downstream. Green or black buoys or posts with a conical cap – keep to the right of these when travelling downstream.
e. Holme – Lock to right of channel.
  Stoke – Lock to left of channel.
  Gunthorpe – Lock to left of channel.
  Hazleford – Lock in middle of river and lock to right of main weir.
  Averham – Long weir on left bank – keep to right hand side of river.
  Newark Nether – Craft heading downstream should wait in the section of the navigation upstream of the railway bridge for the traffic signal instruction to proceed. Craft should not pass beyond these traffic signals until cleared to do so because of the risk of collision. This upper approach is controlled by a closed circuit television.
  Cromwell – Lock to left of channel. River buoyed at this point and large signs erected.

Bye Laws
British Waterways Board's General Canal Bye-Laws 1965 apply and carry a maximum penalty of £100. Under these Bye-Laws all craft should display a current Licence.

Speed Limits
6mph upstream: 8mph downstream.

Do not make a breaking wash, particularly in lock cuttings and canalised or narrow sections.

Reduce speed when:
passing moored craft and fishermen;
passing through sailing or rowing stretches;
passing through water ski-ing zones which are in operation.

Lock Opening Times
Mechanised locks are open from 0600 to 2200 hours Monday to Sunday inclusive. These locks can only be operated by the lock-keepers.

Manual locks are open from 0700 to 1730 hours Monday to Friday and 0700 to 1200 hours on Saturday. Lock-keepers are usually in attendance after normal working hours including Saturday afternoon and Sunday but boaters may operate the locks themselves.

Lock Traffic Lights
These are situated on both sides of the lock entrance and are operated by the lock-keeper when on duty. All boaters must obey the lights when using the locks.

When the lights show RED ONLY – STOP, lock is against you.

When the lights show RED AND GREEN – STAND BY the lock is being prepared.

When the lights show GREEN ONLY – PROCEED, lock is in your favour.

At the manually operated locks there is an additional light:

When the lights show RED WITH SMALL AMBER LIGHT ABOVE – you may operate the lock yourself.

If the lock-keeper has not seen you coming sound a long (4-5 second) blast on your horn.

Dredging Signals
When bucket dredgers are working there are wires across the river and they will display a WHITE disc on the side craft must pass and a RED disc on the side craft must not pass. Do not pass until the WHITE disc is clearly shown.

Tidal Conditions
The Trent is tidal below Cromwell and for those intending to travel beyond Torksey considerable experience of the river is required, or pilotage should be sought from a more experienced boater.

At low tides the river bed dries out in places to leave mud flats. The ebb and flood tides can be used to aid your journey but travelling in opposition to these substantial tidal flows can lead to craft getting into difficulties. BWB lock-keepers, particularly at the tidal locks, will give advice as to the best times to travel.

Flood Conditions
The River Trent is liable to flood at any time of the year and in such circumstances the Board's lock-keepers will give advice on the river conditions, either before or during your journey.

Should you seek advice please be ready to supply information on size and power of your craft and your own experience.

If the conditions are such that it would be too risky to proceed you may be directed to stay in the lock cuttings and moor up.

On rising or falling floodwater you should attend to your mooring ropes regularly.

Fortunately, there is an excellent brochure by J. A. Hutton, *Planning a trip on the Ouse, Trent & Humber,* which goes into considerable detail about such matters, as do the *Sisson's Charts,* published by the Trent Boating Association (please refer to 'Further Reading').

No matter what time you set off, nor from where, unless you are possessed of a very fast, shallow draught vessel, it is more than likely that you will need to wait somewhere near the junction for the young flood. While awaiting a tide there are three choices: Blacktoft Jetty; an anchorage in the Trent; or an anchorage in the Humber.

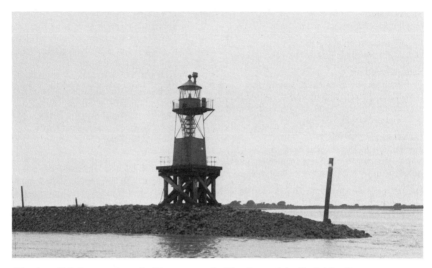

The Apex lighthouse: where the Trent meets the Humber and the Yorkshire Ouse.

BLACKTOFT JETTY
Please refer to the section on this area in the chapter on the River Ouse (p.145).

TRENT ANCHORAGE
This is marked on the chartlet on p.67. At one time it was possible to get out along the channel by the west bank at tide time, and while there is more water there now than there used to be, it is still not possible to use it as an exit. It is important to remember that, after having anchored in the usual spot, it is necessary to back off again so that you cross at the best place; otherwise you stand a serious chance of finding bottom on the sand bank. The holding ground is good, but conditions can be rough, tough and generally quite uncomfortable in as little as Force 4s and 5s, for there is little in the way of high ground to provide anything at all like a lee. But whatever the weather or tide conditions, stout ground tackle and chain of the appropriate calibre are essential if peace of mind is in any way important to you.

HUMBER ANCHORAGE
This is marked on the chartlet on p.67. This potential anchorage lies between the East and West Walker Dyke lights; it is in fairly well protected waters, being under the Lincolnshire lee at least, and has first-rate holding ground. Since the big-ship channel is close, it is essential to drop your hook well away from that channel; that is, towards the south bank. On the chart, it does not look as if there is much room for manoeuvre, but, as in most conversions from chart to reality there is in fact much more to the apparent slight indentation than appears on the page. You will be in no danger from any hazard if you anchor halfway between the channel and the identified bank: vessels will leave you well to starboard and you will not find bottom.

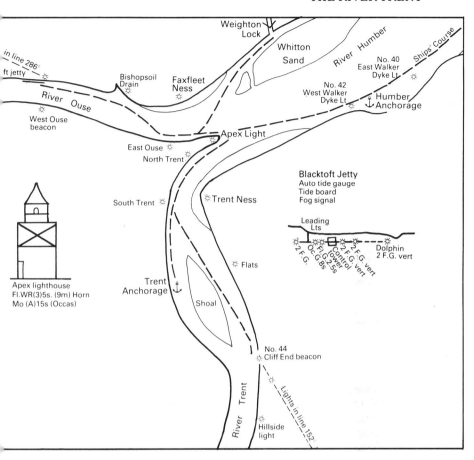

Weighton Lock

Whitton Sand

River Humber

Ships' Course

in line 286 ft jetty

River Ouse

Bishopsoil Drain

Faxfleet Ness

No. 40 East Walker Dyke Lt

No. 42 West Walker Dyke Lt

Humber Anchorage

West Ouse beacon

Apex Light

East Ouse

North Trent

Blacktoft Jetty
Auto tide gauge
Tide board
Fog signal

South Trent

Trent Ness

Leading Lts

2 F.G.

Oc.Fl.G.2.5s

Fl.G.8s

Control tower

2 F.G. vert

2 F.G. vert

Dolphin
2 F.G. vert

Apex lighthouse
Fl.WR(3)5s. (9m) Horn
Mo (A)15s (Occas)

Trent Anchorage

Flats

Shoal

No. 44
Cliff End beacon

River Trent

Hillside light

Lights in line 152

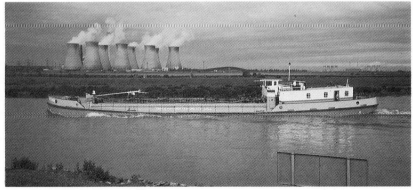

River Trent – typical barge traffic.

However, whichever way you come, and whether or not you need or intend to anchor, you will sooner or later be wanting to identify the Apex lighthouse. In this area, it is certainly not to be considered as a light that is hid under a bushel; indeed, it is more to be likened to a beacon that stands out as a goodly deed in a naughty world, although it does so somewhat starkly (and a bit like a hutch) and gauntly . . . and while you may not need to run either gauntlets or legs at a great rate of knots, nevertheless it is necessary to keep enough power on in order to retain steerage control in what can only be described as tricky and fickle but lusty and doughty waters. The channel runs very close to the banks on the flanks of the Apex peninsula, that is, by the east Ouse and north Trent beacons respectively, and for those two half-mile stretches, there is probably the deepest water to be found in the whole of the northeast waterways between Boston and Ripon. A distance of ½-¾ cable off avoids all hazards; the main ones being the stones of the training walls (very well marked by posts) and the shoal banks out in the river by Faxfleet Ness and Trent Ness, both of which are marked (occasional! and conspicuous!), at times when you should be sure to avoid them, by the regular congregations of food-seeking birds that gather together there. In fact, it is a veritable confluence at the confluence, and thoroughly deserves a special note: 'DANGER: Birds at work – Look out for Shoals.'

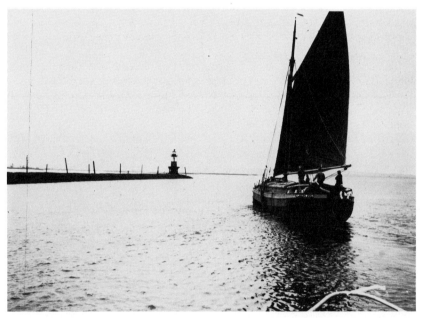

The Humber Keel & Sloop Society's *Amy Howson* sailing down the Trent.

And looking out for shoals is what the next stretch, the actual entry into the tideway of the Trent proper, is all about: namely, finding, and keeping, the shallow channel that crosses the Trent from the west bank to the east bank. There are leading marks and lights on the east (the Burton-upon-Stather) side and they are to be kept in line not only with themselves but also with the south Trent beacon on the Apex peninsula. It is important to remember that if you are navigating on the ebb, it will tend to set you down river and on to the ground of the Trent Ness; and if you are working the flood, especially if it is the young flood with little water anywhere around, it will tend to set you on the notorious sandbank that occupies (in terms of drying or shoaling) very nearly fifty acres. The Admiralty Pilot notes that the tidal stream can exceed six knots.

The chartlet for Trent Falls (on p.67) is not intended for navigation. Intending skippers should obtain up-to-date charts for the area from the ABP offices in Hull. There are two charts: *Spurn to Barton Haven; Barton Haven to Burton Stather*. They are essential for cruising in the area of Trent Falls. I have often been offered a pair of charts that, according to their proud owners, 'have only been used for a couple of years' and would give me all the information I needed 'at half the price!' Since the channels vary so frequently (and often dramatically, as the sketch map on p.226 shows for the Humber, with Trent End also in contention with its nesses and banks) it is important to have the very latest information. ABP Hull will send you the charts and all the relevant corrections through the post. A telephone call will get the charts and an invoice to you; and, if you need more up-to-date information about possible changes to markers or floats, a telephone call will also give you that. The *Spurn to Barton* is published annually before Easter, and the *Barton to Burton* is published every two months.

There are a few more special points about the Trent that are worth noting: while the ABP chart of the upper river covers the stretch from Trent Falls to the Waddington light on the west bank, their survey vessels keep an eye on the river much further up than that; in fact, the responsibility of the ABP Hull harbour master extends to the south side of the stone bridge in Gainsborough. The official VHF radio channel up to Keadby Bridge is 12, but many skippers of the barges and coasters that ply frequently in these waters tend to use 6, (and this is the regular channel further up the river) and also to change to 8, 9 or 10 as impulse, traffic or a wish not to be monitored may dictate. All the locks up the river work VHF channels 16 and 74 and will, some with enthusiasm and others with reluctance, work channel 6 for those skippers without 74.

In terms of finding the best water, the general rule is the predictable one regarding rivers with any kind of flow: the deepest water is on the outside of the bends; and the 'ness' is to be found on the inside. However, the 'inside' can often extend with gently sloping sand, mud and silt to well past the middle of the river. It is always worthwhile keeping a weather eye open for those changes apparent on the surface water that indicate where the deeps end and the shallows start. In addition, just to complicate matters, there are quite a few vessels using the Trent (and this can also apply to the Ouse and the Humber) that are constrained by their draught or are trying to negotiate tricky bends and as a result are to be found on the 'wrong' side of the road. It is important to give way to such vessels as they will not be able to pass you 'port to port', nor will they try. A listening watch on the radio will bring news of vessels in the vicinity proposing to pass one another 'green to green' and that should be enough to alert the cruising skipper to watch out. A working knowledge of sound signals, and a willingness to use and respond to them, will also be of great assistance. I have always found that the skippers of working craft on this river are more than ready to co-operate with cruising vessels, provided they can see there is a readiness on the part of leisure-folk to participate in a similar vein.

Once upon a time, the Trent eagre (aegir, aegre, eager or bore) was a marvel and a wonder; a monster wall of implacable water making what seemed like a royal progress; that is, of Neptune seated on a hippocampus, overwhelming all before him. That is how I remember it as a boy being taken to witness its advance up the river from the banks just below Keadby bridge. That was more than fifty years ago and since then there have been training walls, draining schemes and massively engined coasters churning their way to Gainsborough, with the result that it is now little more than a token reminder of its former glorious but threatening self. Nevertheless, as I have had it put to me: 'It is not to be encountered broadsides on, standing in a dinghy.' If there is any chance that you are going to be involved in its path, make sure you take it straight on if under way, and if moored up slacken off your lines to give three or four feet extra slack especially on your head rope. Nowadays, the eagre seldom exceeds a couple of feet, but in those times gone by it did get up to more than seven. This quite unusual and remarkable phenomenon is created by a combination of long, strong winds and an abnormally high spring tide. The already high tide is further impelled by the wind behind it until, as it floods up the narrowing river, it becomes the amazing surge that has been described as 'the forerunner of the Kraken waking' – and, most alarming to an impressionable child, it made a sound like that of the Titans organising themselves for battle.

While cruising the Trent, I met quite a few people who said they hoped I would take 'the bogey' out of the Trent, and they were not talking of any eagre. It is true that with some cruising folk the Trent has a reputation for being a harsh master, and having once had a slightly off-putting experience on it, they avoid it like the plague. I know that many newcomers to the river who have left Torksey a little on the late side for Keadby, or who have been too taken by sight-seeing to make sure they were not losing ground, have been quite happily going down the last few miles to the motorway bridge on a quiet ebb when they have been stopped 'dead in their tracks' (as one of them described it) simply by the change of conditions as the flood took them unawares. To change, unexpectedly, from a flow going with you at (say) two knots to one that is against you at (say) three knots, means that while your speed through the water remains the same (say three knots) your speed over the ground will drop from five knots to an awe-inspiring standstill. However, any such shock and displeasure experienced must surely be attributable to the skipper rather than to any 'bogey' of the Trent. 'Be prepared' must be the watchword.

But, 'Be prepared' for what? Above Torksey, I must confess, there is little to prompt alarms or excursions, for it can never be said that the stretch up to Cromwell from Torksey Cut can be a pretender to the crown of hobgoblin, phantom, bugbear or bugaboo. In any case, most boaters tend to cruise around those parts in small flotillas so that most potential snags are well covered and the tricky bits (if that is what they must be called) well known to at least one member of the group. Below Torksey, however, the situation is different: although there is, in fact, no 'bogey' of any kind to be encountered on the Trent, the truth is that the river below Torksey should not be attempted by craft, crew or skippers that are not equipped to cruise The Wash or other coastal waters. I am of the opinion that the Trent should be treated as a small seaway: once that precaution has been taken, the waterway can take its place with all the others that must be treated with respect if they are to be properly appreciated and enjoyed.

(But, I have seen too many 15' GRP cruisers with, typically, 4h.p. outboards, two parents, two children under five and often cat or dog to boot, with no buoyancy aid, radio or anchor, shoot out of Keadby Lock on a spring flood like corks out of a bottle, and without as much as a by-your-leave, or a moment's wait for the keeper to give the OK, not to feel that serious warnings are in order. What will rid the river of any 'bogey' is appropriate preparation: one would not think of going on a coastal cruise without some relevant experience, proper navigation aids, decent life-jackets, and sound cleats, ropes, chain and anchor. There is no reason to treat the Trent any differently.)

So, after all the precautions, warnings and preparations, we can get started: and the beginning of the Trent peregrination is much more dramatic than the next stretch which is pretty bleak and unchanging until you reach Burton-upon-Stather. It is quite a scenic vision after all the muddy monotony, and the trees and cliffs do their best to welcome you to one of the best-known and best-loved of Scunthorpe's picnic and courting spots: Burton Hills. It is not long however, before any glimpses of scenery have been lost in favour of hundreds of metres of commercial quays and jetties at Kingsferry (Burton), Flixborough, Neap House, Grove Wharf, Gunness and Keadby, and, with the sudden and unexpected upsurge of traffic due to the coal dispute of 1984-5, a considerable increase in the number of ships of considerable tonnage using the river hereabouts. There is certainly plenty to look at, but it does not consist of the Trent's best scenery at this stage in the exploration. In general, the river follows a definite pattern as it flows through the Trent valley: woods, hills, jetties and most other items that are of any passing interest to the spectator all appear on the east banks; to the west there is little but flats and flatness all the way.

One of the exceptions to that rule, is the jetty, lock and folk-community that go to make up the conglomerate of Keadby. Once upon a time, there was a ferry to Gunness; a packet to Kingston-upon-Hull; a doctor who used to cross the river in something like a coracle; a power station that damn near devoured the native spirit of the indigenes; and a constant procession of traffic by road, rail and water that kept the place thriving well beyond its natural time. And even now, it may, from some angles, seem to be dead; but there is no chance that it is going to lie down without a struggle, for those who have remained carry within them the unique genes that enabled the antediluvian citizens of the Isle of Axholme to surve *sui generis* when all around them succumbed to horde after invading horde. Keadby is not a place to be taken at its face value, or, if it is, then the best face to consider is that of the King George bascule bridge: although the railway station it serves is now called 'Althorpe', it used to be known as 'Keadby and Althorpe'; and the bridge has never been known by any name other than Keadby Bridge.

When I was a child, that bridge was a wonder of my world. It carried pedestrians, cyclists, cars, buses and lorries without hint of strain, stress or even reaction; however, when the Doncaster-to-Grimsby goods train passed at the same time as extra-heavy transporters from the local iron and steelworks then its frame would shudder – and so would mine. The bridge itself was to me a source of fear and delight – in almost equal proportions – and when it hinged upwards, opening for the river traffic that it then still accommodated, I was transfixed as it reared menacingly towards its final inclination.

The bridge is still a wondrous thing, and steaming under it can still arouse a sense of awe; but, like its possibly eponymous neighbour, its past is more impressive than its present, and you must persevere if you are to find the pearls that abound by street and stream.

More germane is the matter of the lock and getting into the canal. As few know, the jetty just above the lock does offer a reasonable alternative to locking in (if you merely want to stop over for a tide and then press on up river). It also means that you can get away much earlier on the tide than if you were actually

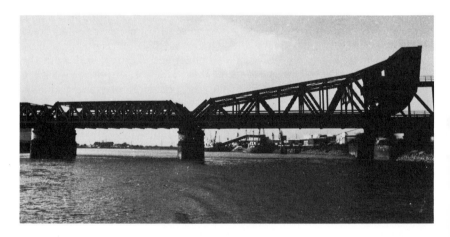

The King George Bridge at Keadby – no more to lift again. The deepest water is to be found under the old lifting arch (to the right in picture).

inside. Craft drawing up to two metres will not bottom by the lock end of the jetty, even on the lowest of neaps. Once or twice I have tried to gain permission from one of the coasters that regularly use the downstream jetty to lay alongside, but usually skippers and crew alike tend to suffer from that deaf-to-yachtsmen affliction that totally incapacitates them; until you meet them shoresides on the bank of the canal when they may suddenly come alive, alert and co-operative in their attempts to seduce you into a snap purchase of their contraband goods. I have never even succeeded in raising them let alone gaining their consent or help; however, Henry Irving claims that he has always found them helpful – but then, the *William McCann* not only draws 'plenty water' but also pulls 'plenty strings'.

The actual entry into the lock can be a bit tricky: just like Selby and West Stockwith locks, it gives directly on to the tideway, and that always causes problems. If coming downstream with the ebb, the routine is to pass the lock, round up and then make diagonally for the upriver stonework knuckle. Once there, a nudge of power and a gentle (firm but gentle) turn on the wheel will nose the vessel in. Coming upstream with the flood, the routine is similar: pass the lock, round up and then make for a holding position parallel to the upstream jetty (or any vessel that might be in possession). With a little luck, one of the lock-keepers (or a colleague) will be there to take a line from you and assist your vessel round the bend. If there is no-one ashore to help, a crew member can take a rope up the jetty ladder and lead you in. If you are single-handed, at least you have been warned, for the chances are that the flood will pin you against the timbers – so plenty of sound fenders and stout ropes will be needed. If all this sounds just too hairy or strenuous, simply tie up and await high water. (There are many 'knowing' skippers who do this to make sure of an extra hour or two's time for drinking in the local hostelries.)

For an easy entry, you need a neap tide, plenty of water above the mud spits at the entrance (see p.74-5) and no more than two coasters (with both on the lower jetty). Keadby is the door to the canal system that leads to Thorne, Doncaster, Sheffield, Leeds, Wakefield, Selby and Goole. However, easy entry or not, Keadby is not a place to be missed for anything but the most dire emergency or sombre cause, for, once moored up, you will begin to appreciate the delights that surround you. You can hardly avoid a good crack and confabulation of what Pope calls 'the feast of reason and the flow of the soul'. Firstly, there is the team of lock-keepers who, to a man, are undisputably, incorrigibly and indefatigably characterful. You may not at first throw be able to draw from them their insight into the nature of infinity, the world, the flesh or the devil; indeed, it is just possible, due to the exigencies of the human condition, that you may find it a slow process to extract the time of the next flood – but they are men to be pursued with perseverance, and, in the fullness of time, you will discover that you are, if not actually cosseted, then at least well favoured. Also special when it comes to any kind of discourse, debate or deliberation, is the 'maister' of Keadby Marine Engineering, George Trevithic. He is no ancient mariner, but he can certainly hold you with his glittering eye

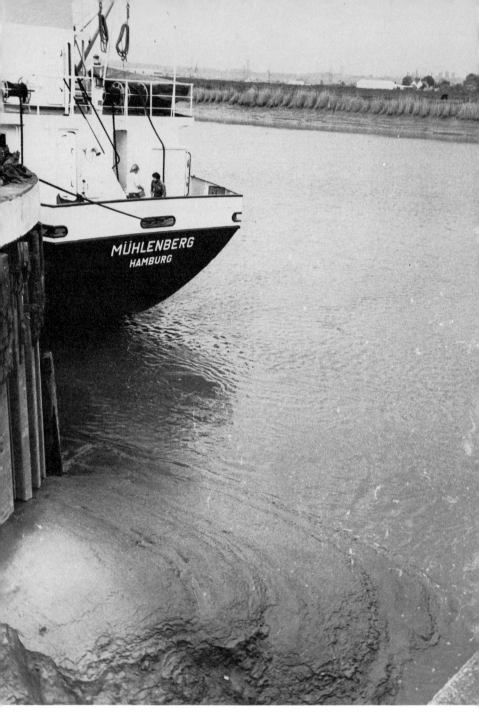

The entrance to the lock at Keadby, showing the two problems likely to be encountered: the outstanding mud spits; and the likelihood of coasters.

KEADBY LOCK

BWB Keadby Lock,
Trentside,
Keadby,
Scunthorpe, South Humberside
☎ Scunthorpe (0724) 782205
VHF channels 16 and 74.

Restricting dimensions 77′8″ x 21′10″
Rise and fall (tidal)
Hand operated •
Keeper operated •
Facilities nearby

⚓ 🚾 ⛽

🐟 Keadby Marine Ltd – above lock
(0724) 782302. Diesel only.
🛢 Friendship (0724) 782243
S General stores
✉ 2 minutes walk
♪ 200 yards from lock
⚓

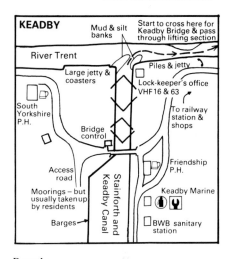

KEADBY

Mud & silt banks

Start to cross here for Keadby Bridge & pass through lifting section

River Trent

Large jetty & coasters

Piles & jetty

Lock-keeper's office VHF 16 & 63

South Yorkshire P.H.

To railway station & shops

Bridge control

Friendship P.H.

Access road

Stainforth and Keadby Canal

Keadby Marine

Moorings – but usually taken up by residents

BWB sanitary station

Barges

Remarks
See also notes on p.107.

KEADBY

Trent Falls 10 miles
West Stockwith 12 miles
Cromwell Lock 43 miles
Thorne 10 miles

Moorings
There are two main jetties outside the lock: one immediately downstream of the entrance and one above it. The one above it is sometimes available to pleasure craft; and even if occupied, it may be that the commercial skipper will be co-operative and take your lines. Downstream of the entrance is to be avoided by all pleasure craft; and upstream you should notify the lock-keeper of your presence; just in case he hasn't seen you arrive! Inside the lock (after the huge doors and the road swing bridge) there are moorings on each side of the canal. In season, they tend to be very crowded, and often there are queues alongside the water and sanitary station – sometimes rafted up.

Facilities nearby

🐟 Only in the village
S (must be described as 'limited')
⚓ ✕ ● ♪ 🛢 ⛽

Remarks
The entrance to the lock can be complicated by the rate of flow of the flood; the two mud spits that strike out from the entrance knuckles; and the presence of a number of coasters, sometimes making sight lines and the approach run tricky . . . especially if they happen to have their screws turning as they are known to do.

The rise and fall can achieve up to sixteen feet: Stout gear is mandatory.

and enthral you with his remembrances of things past. His eye for a piece of common copper or plain brass is just as bright as if he is contemplating a marvel of steam-powered magic driving some mighty Wurlitzer at a fair-ground reunion. Not only that, he and his son are more likely than almost anyone else within a radius of fifty miles to be able to diagnose your condition, make useful suggestions, put them into effective practice; and, as an extra bonus, 'just happen to have' that obsolete, impossible-to-obtain, spare part lurking in one of their many and varied premises. They sell diesel and gas.

If your need for fuel is of a different kind, there are three public houses within arm-lifting reach of the moorings: the Mariners Arms, the South Yorkshire and the Friendship. They are all of interest and are all quite different in style and clientele. It is necessary to visit them all at least once to make up your mind which one is for you. I have never noticed all that much difference in the way they keep their beer, but the real ale buffs say that only one of them is really worth a visit.

I have a high regard for the settlement of Keadby and its collection of personable persons (although you must be warned that the shopkeepers do not like accepting cheques even backed by bankers' cards, so there must be some rogues about) and always try to spend a good few days there just mooching around seeing what is what, and how it has changed – which is usually not at all. The last time I stayed there I got involved in an experience that tellingly demonstrated the kind of trying life and times that the lock-keepers can have. Having to wait for neaps to pass (it had been a droughty year and there seemed to be no fresh water in the Trent at all, with the result that neither Stockwith nor Torksey could get me in) I spent a few days lending a hand to Walt and Derek, the duty lock-keepers, whenever there was a 'pen'.

On one occasion, the lock was almost crammed, and the boats were all manned by novices except for the know-all wife of a know-all skipper. Both Derek and I had tried to keep her out of the various troubles she seemed intent upon wreaking on herself and on each attempt we had been rewarded with an earful of arrogant, aggressive abuse. I decided that retreat was the better part of action and so returned to *Valcon* and the moorings. Shortly after, they all steamed past. In the vanguard, of course, was the offensive boat-wife. Suddenly she started to point at *Valcon* and me and to shout violently at her husband as if I were not there. I heard the words 'that chap Bowskill' followed by something about *Motor Boat and Yachting* , and that was enough for me: I disappeared below. However, that was to no avail for after about fifteen minutes the self-same female was assertively knocking on the windows of the wheelhouse.

Without the slightest bit of attention to what I might have felt, she hoisted herself aboard and started to berate me. It later became clear that she was trying to apologise in her own inimitable way, but it came out like a tirade: 'I'm sorry I lost my rag back there. What can I say? You didn't seem to be doing what I wanted, so I thought 'bloody hell', but it was a genuine mistake. You see, I would never have shouted at you like that if I had known you were somebody; you know! I just took it for granted you were the lock-keeper'!!! The exclamation marks are mine. No wonder some lock-keepers adopt a cool and passive manner; and no wonder some of them lose their cool from time to time and become a bit more active.

If you let the lock-keepers know your draught, speed and destination, they will advise you what time to leave the lock to proceed up river. Once out of the lock, you should keep to starboard going upstream until you reach the most

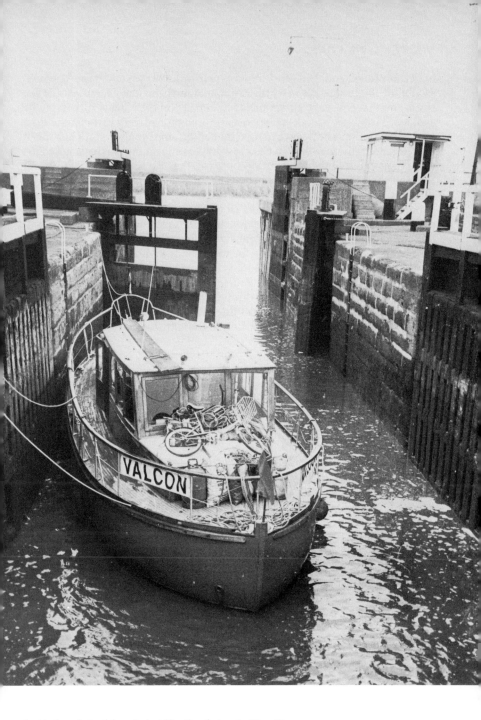

Inside the substantial sea-lock at Keadby, facing the River Trent.

noticeable house and then gently cross over in order to pass under the 'opening' section of the bridge. (It is worth taking a look at the low- water state of the river, and that will show an advancing mud bank on the other side that is to be avoided. However, unless you are over 6′ draught and very early on the tide, which you couldn't be if you had been in the lock since you wouldn't have been able to get out, there will be no need to worry about running out of water.) This is the first of four road bridges below Newark; the next is the M180, the second the stone bridge at Gainsborough, and the third, a toll bridge, at Dunham. Of the next riverside communities: Butterwick, Owston Ferry – but ferry long gone, Wildsworth, Gunthorpe and East and West Stockwith even, little can be seen from water level. There is not much to do, to see or to complain about in this stretch; there is little that will exhaust or threaten from the river, and in no time at all you will be approaching the wide bends in the river that mark West Stockwith. The lock-keeper will be watching out for you, for even if you haven't been in touch with him yourself (either on VHF or land line) the Keadby contingent will have rung through to let him know what kind of 'delivery' he is likely to expect on the next tide. The first real sign that you are near the lock is the entrance to the River Idle on the west bank, not far downstream from the canal.

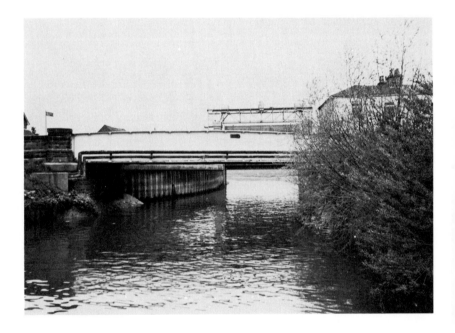

The entrance to the River Idle from the River Trent.

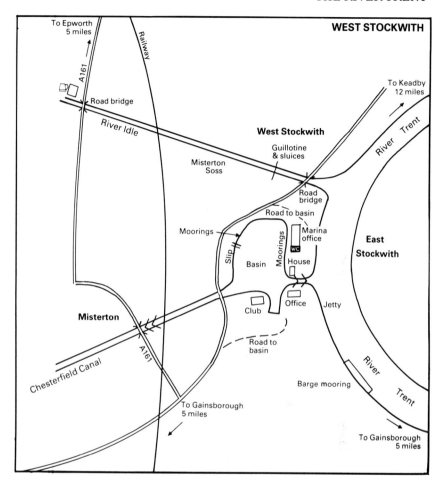

Getting into the lock at West Stockwith requires something of a similar manoeuvre to that used at Keadby; dependent upon the state of the tides and your direction at the time, make for the knuckle of the upstream wall if on the ebb, rounding up if you need to and make for the jetty on the upstream wall if on the flood (also rounding up if necessary). You are more likely to find a collection of onlooking helpers here than at any other lock on the Trent; the place seems a veritable magnet at tide times. The main difficulty is likely to arise if you are trying to negotiate the entrance when there is a strong spring flood running; in which case (after consulting the lock-keeper) you may think it best to hang on outside for a time until the stream loses some of its vigour.

WEST STOCKWITH LOCK

British Waterways Board
West Stockwith Lock,
Misterton,
Doncaster,
S. Yorks.
☎ Gainsborough (0427) 890204
VHF channels 16 and 74

Restricting dimensions 72' x 17'6" x 6' (depth of basin).
Rise and fall (tidal)
Keeper operated ●
Facilities nearby

⚓ ᵂᶜ 🛢

🏪 1½ miles
S 2 miles
✉ ¾ mile
☎ ¾ mile

Remarks

1. The lock will be operation for periods of 7 hours per tide, from 2½ hours before to 4½ hours after high water.
2. For passage through the lock between 0800 hours and 2200 hours boaters are requested to give as much advance notice as possible.
3. For passage through the lock between 2200 hours and 0800 hours the lock must be booked at least 24 hours in advance. Ansaphone facilities are available in the absence of the lock-keeper or his relief.

In addition to the above the lock-keeper will be on duty from 1st April to 30th September on Saturday, Sunday and Bank Holidays between 0800 and 2000 hours. During this period he will be available for general enquiries, slipping and licences.

There is a tide gauge just outside the lock, and the keeper advises that if you presume that there is one foot less water than is indicated you will not go far wrong. Ironically, more boats get into trouble by trying to get into the lock when there is insufficient water than through any other factor. I have seen pictures of keel boats having gone aground in the cut and nearby, and the sight is not a pretty one; in fact, one boat was a complete write off. Because of the flood walls, the keeper cannot always have full view of what is going on in the river; so, if you find that, for any reason, you are better standing off in the main channel of the river, just give a single blast on the horn and he should appear. As he rightly points out: 'No-one likes those skippers who blast away from five miles off, but there are also those who are far too hesitant in using their whistles. It's much better to give a blow than to do the wrong thing and risk life and limb.'

Once inside West Stockwith Basin, all kinds of delights await you: there is the well-run lock (office, workshop, yard and cottage); a yacht club that could not be more friendly and welcoming but without in any way being pushy; Milethorne Marina and West Stockwith Yacht Services who offer a service that is surprisingly well orientated for sea-going craft, with a chandlery that deserves not only patronage but also carefully considered digging and delving, for it is comprehensively stockpiled with a range of merchandise that, at one and the same time, manages to be useful, sensible, intriguing and idiosyncratic; and an array of boats covering a much wider spectrum than one might expect in such a basin.

Away from the lock, there is the Chesterfield Canal and the River Idle (both of which are dealt with later in this chapter) and, of course, the village itself. There is an East Stockwith and the two halves gaze somewhat disconsolately at one another across the river that, in that area, tempts no-one to think of crossing it except by the bridges that are Gainsborough and Keadby distant. West

WEST STOCKWITH

Trent Falls 22 miles
Cromwell Lock 31 miles

Moorings

BWB and marina moorings within the basin; with more available just out of the basin on either side of the Chesterfield Canal through the small road bridge. If you draw around 6', you will need local advice to find you an appropriate 'hole'.

Marina

Milethorne Marine, West Stockwith Yacht Basin, West Stockwith, Doncaster.
☎ Gainsborough (0427) 890450.

This is not a mammoth operation, but they do provide, as they say, 'all marine sales and service'; in any case, they have their eyes on the Trent's horizon and are planning and preparing for a future they see as expanding. You will be treated as an individual by a team of individuals; and the place and its environment are both so intriguingly peculiar and enigmatic (and I use both words advisedly) that you will find yourself tempted to stay longer than you planned. Boatyard facilities are also provided by the same management, with slip for craft up to 50'.

Club

West Stockwith Yacht Club Ltd., The Club House, The Yacht Basin, West Stockwith, Doncaster. ☎ Gainsborough (0427) 890673. Here you will find another variation of the West Stockwith special hospitality: on one occasion when I was cruising very late in the year and the weather was northeast-midlands awful, they opened up the premises late at night just so that I could make a phone call; they didn't even try to sell me a drink, in fact, insisted on giving me one 'on the house'. Long may they thrive.

Facilities

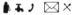

S (2 miles)

Remarks

There are two special factors: the entrance to the lock, being straight off the river can be tricky; and there is not a lot of mooring space for craft of 6'. The best spot is just round the corner to the left immediately after leaving the lock: that is, in the basin and close to the club house. If at all in doubt, have a word with the lock-keeper before you arrive; he may be able to find you a small corner.

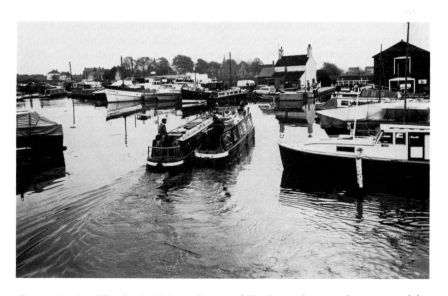

The canal basin at West Stockwith is usually pretty full and pretty busy – and a pretty spot it is.

Stockwith straggles along the riverside road towards Gunthorpe, Lady Croft and Hemdyke, but not really properly getting into its stride until after the River Idle. Then there is the first pub; with an exceedingly young and lively clientele, that shows quite clearly that not all our youth are drifting away from the land. There used to be one immediately opposite the lock basin, but it has not opened its doors to thirsty travellers for some long time now.

Even if you are not proposing to cruise either the River Idle or the Chesterfield Canal, West Stockwith is a place to visit and to linger over, so don't ever steam by unless you have to.

Just above Stockwith, on the starboard hand going upstream, there is a jetty which often plays host to a barge. I have been told on a number of occasions that it is safe to moor there and that a 6' vessel will stay afloat alongside the barge. However, I have not as yet actually met anyone who has positively done it, and I am always keenly aware of the sharpness of the bend and the consequential risk there must be should any barge or coaster bound for Gainsborough find itself in difficulty when negotiating it. I am sure that no pleasure cruiser should think of using it except in the direst of emergencies.

The five miles from West Stockwith to Gainsborough are straightforward both from a scenic and a navigational point of view. The first noticeable sign that you are near the town is Gleadell's Wharf (on the east bank) and the huge bend that sweeps round almost 270 degrees before recovering its sense of direction (to the west). This area opposite the outlying community of Morton is prone to flooding, and at big high waters can present a confusing acreage that demands keen eyes to pick out the slender beacons that go to delineate the banks. Under normal circumstances, the river and the deep water channel are obvious, and the only hazard you may possibly meet (and that is most unlikely) will have been caused, in all likelihood, by a congestion of commercial traffic. I have passed through Gainsborough fairly often and have never found the traffic to be anything but helpful to pleasure vessels and very quick indeed to help them out of trouble. Indeed, I once witnessed a bit of neat and speedy rope work that prevented a narrow boat going broadsides into the stone bridge; and that was thanks to a watchful crew on a foreign coaster.

Sadly, there is no mooring in Gainsborough that can properly be recommended to pleasure craft. Some skippers take their chances along what I assess as 'doubtful' jetties, and others have lain alongside a coaster. I feel that the rate and rise and fall of the stream, together with the paucity of moorings that are suitable for pleasure craft make Gainsborough a non-starter when it comes to finding a stopping place. There is great scope for development along the riverside in this town, and it is to the shame of the riparian city fathers that they have done so little for so long, and have let the waterside so badly deteriorate that it is virtually unusable except for its trading wharfs. As for the rest: it is dilapidated, uncared for and ignored; making Gainsborough into a positive jewel of a place in a negative, tarnished setting.

There is another jewel about ten miles up the river; but before we get to that miniature, there are some of the trickiest stretches of the Trent to be

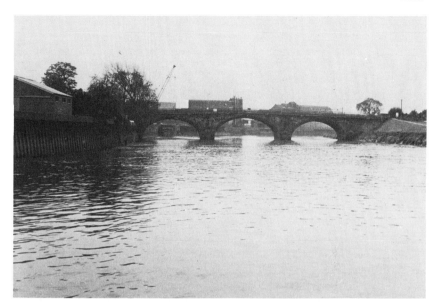

The stone bridge, Gainsborough, where authority changes from Associated British Ports, Hull to British Waterways Board, Nottingham.

negotiated, starting with the stone bridge at the south end of the town. Here, on the south face, is where the responsibility of the harbour master of the Humber ceases and where the authority of the BWB takes over; and here also is where it is appropriate to approach with caution if your air draught is near three metres. Since the river is still tidal at this point and there can be considerable fresh water coming down, it is by no means an exact science to assess the possible headroom that may be available. Other things being equal (which, of course, they seldom are) there should be a headroom of 9′ at MHWS, when there is a rise of 10′. If you are in any doubt at all, it must be the best course of action (when going with the flood, which most skippers will be doing) to turn well before the bridge and gently stem the tide so that you reach the bridge at a dead slow speed, stern first. Should things not be in your favour, you will at least have the advantage of being able to keep out of trouble without any difficulty.

After the bridge the river once more goes in for some huge bends right up to Torksey. The first is just outside Gainsborough and seems to go on for ages; and then there are more past the power station and also at Knaith, where there is a well known landmark: the pseudo-half-timbered mansion set well back in the trees. There is also a quaint boathouse to catch the eye. It is the next two bends that require special attention: Littleborough and Marton (also known as Trent Port). Unless you are navigating near low water with a draught of 6′, you should not encounter problems if you keep within the channel (please refer to the chartlet on p.84.)

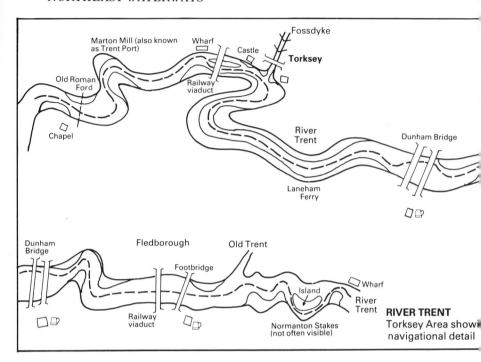

RIVER TRENT
Torksey Area showi
navigational detail

After the pumping station that marks the end of the Marton Bend it is not far to the fuel-oil jetty just before Torksey railway viaduct, where you should take the port arch going upstream. Immediately after comes the village on the east bank, well marked by the remains of the castle and, a little more upstream just by the canal cut, the pumping station on the bend. Frequently, there are tugs and barges working in the area. On the west bank there is a tide gauge; towards the east side of the river, there is shoal ground running from the viaduct for 3 to 4 cables upstream, and it is wise not to cross over to the Torksey side until well clear. Indeed, there is no hazard in tending to keep to starboard until Torksey Cut opens up. Don't try cutting corners on the way into the Cut, for there can be silt and mud spits reaching out quite a distance from both banks. It is best to open up the Cut from a central course in the river and then take a straight, central line in. The channel lies in the middle and unless there has been an exceptionally dry year, craft of up to 6′ will be able to reach the staging just before the road bridge and the lock at any state of the tide. The wooden staging is in good order and provides an excellent waiting berth for the lock, or for overnight. A vessel drawing 6′ will stay afloat at all times provided it stays away from the bridge end, where there can be no more than 3′. When a laden barge passes the entrance to the Cut at a good speed, there can be a surge reaching right to the lock, and it can be powerful enough to strain or even part ropes. On a neap tide, with the lock gates open, compensating precautions should be taken even in the lock itself.

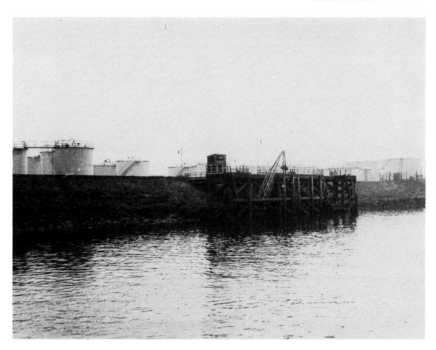

The fuel jetty just below Torksey viaduct.

Torksey Castle.

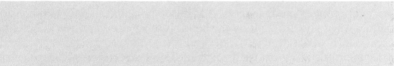

TORKSEY LOCK

British Waterways Board,
Torksey Lock,
Torksey,
Lincoln
☎ Torksey (042771) 202
VHF channels 16 and 74

Restricting dimensions 81'5" x 16'6" x 6'10" (varies)
Torksey to Lincoln   75' x 15'3" x 5'
Lincoln to Boston   75' x 15'3" x 4'6"
Rise and fall   (tidal)
Keeper operated   •
Facilities nearby

⚓ 🚻 🗗 ♪

Torksey is a miniature, superficially offering very little to engage any passer-by, but after deeper penetration you will find that it is possessed of an unlikely charisma and that its populace can be as quaint as they are astute and as dyed-in-the-wool as they are forward looking, for there are plenty who combine a genuine and altruistic hospitality with a keen eye not only for the main chance but also for any kind of chance that happens to promise financial reward. I think that Torksey can only be found wanting in the commonplace. (For maps and further detail, please see p.56)

After Torksey, there comes a series of racks, shoals and stakes before Cromwell Lock is reached. The channel does not change very much and the chartlet on p.84 shows the pattern between Marton and Normanton. There are only two contenders for any doubt at all: the big bend after Torksey power station; and Fledborough railway viaduct. The exact location of the channel around the bend is still subject to conjecture; some skippers prefer the outside of the inside, while others prefer the inside of the outside. However, there is full agreement that it does not run on the outside of the outside, nor on the inside of the inside. My personal experience after a number of encounters with the ground (harmless mud) suggests that it is to be found slightly to the inside of middle when you are right on the bend. It must also be added that, on those occasions, it was at dead low water and there had been drought conditions for three months and *Valcon* needs six feet. 'Local experts' are also divided about which arch to use when passing under the Fledborough viaduct; some use the left arch when going upstream, while others use the right one. I have tried both, and sounded the area as well, but have found little difference. More information can be gleaned from the Trent Boating Association's *Handbook for the Trent*.

The stretch of river from Torksey to Cromwell consists of 16 miles of scenery which gets slowly better the further upstream you cruise; and at the same time, the tide begins to lose most of its sting. Some of the views that are afforded in this region are typical of Nottinghamshire at its best; and, all in all, it is an extremely pleasant leg from the diminutive lock at Torksey to the massive construction and formidable weir that go to make up the tidal/flood barrier that is Cromwell. Its name may refer more to historical events than to eponymous characteristics, but there is no denying that the place is just about as Cromwellian and sombre as it could be. Happily, there is naught that is Cromwellian about Cliff Fields, the keeper of Cromwell. While he is neither draconian nor stentorian (and at times he must be sorely tempted to be both) he will get you

CROMWELL LOCK

British Waterways Board
Cromwell Lock,
North Muskham,
Nr. Newark,
Notts. NG23 6HX
☎ Newark (0636) 821213
VHF channels 16 and 74

Restricting dimensions   187′ x 30′
Rise and fall   (tidal)
Mechanised   ●
Keeper operated   ●
Facilities nearby
⚓

Remarks
Upstream of Cromwell, the navigation channel is 6′ deep and this dimension may be more relevant than lock dimensions.

Practical maximum dimensions of craft between Gainsborough and Nottingham 140′ x 18′6″ x 6′

Hours of operation:
Mon. 0600-2100 hours
Tues.-Sun. 0600-2200 hours
Breaks from 1200-1230 and 1730-1800.

in and out at the right times and in the right way and proper manner, often in spite of your own best but ill-conceived plans, and your even worse executed efforts.

Timing is 'of the essence' when leaving Cromwell and will, to a certain extent, be governed by your draught, speed and destination; and if you are wise it will be totally governed by the lock-keeper's advice regarding the expectation of water, since the rise and fall of tidal waters can be as little as 4″ (with an ebb that lingers for all of eleven hours) and the head of fresh as likely as not to reach 4′ (on the day you want to leave, of course, Sod's Law being what it is) it is well worthwhile listening to those who know the ways of the Trent. Since there is nowhere on the tidal stretches (except the 3 locked entrances at Torksey, Stockwith and Keadby) where you can possibly moor in any kind of safety, it is only sensible to keep as many aspects of this river on your side as you can and working the tides properly is an essential one.

The lock itself is a sombre thing; it is possessed of a large chamber with deep sides, and can look, on a dark, dank day, very threatening. If the pit itself is dark and awesome, the nearby weir vies with it for effect and impact, for it is wide, brilliant and rushing, and in the past has dealt swiftly and mercilessly with those who have approached it not wisely but too closely. Nowadays, the weir is well marked and there is no risk at all of getting too close to it by chance although we can all fall victim to accident or carelessness. It is the lock that is of interest to cruising folk, marking the entry to the non-tidal waters that are more than 50 miles away from the mouth of the Trent, which is somewhat idiosyncratically placed not at Trent Mouth at all, but at Trent Falls (or as it is often called, just to confuse the newcomer even more, Trent End). Here you will find the dramatic demarcation between the shallow tidal reaches upstream of Torksey and, what is for most of the rest of its journey up to Nottingham, a fairly lush experience with deepish, clean water all the way.

A little way up the river, and about half way to Newark, is the tiny village of North Muskham, where there is a staging platform conveniently placed for the local pub, the Newcastle Arms. (Vessels of more than 4′ are advised not to try and moor there. I have been advised that the bottom could be foul, but have not been able to verify.) The village itself is a pleasant, quiet little place but with all basic domestic facilities. Across the river is another equally quiet community, Holme: this is even smaller and with fewer facilities than Muskham. There is no proper access from the river for Holme.

The next stopping place proper is Newark, where there are two locks: Nether and Town. Nether is, as you would expect, the lower of the two and is situated on the outskirts of the town; Town, equally expectedly, is almost central. They are both mechanised, manned, on the phone and VHF radio. There is also a BWB yard here, and the old lock now forms moorings for small craft and a dry dock, which can also be used by the public. Arrangements are made through the BWB office and a charge is made.

Newark is riddled with monuments to its history and its heritage; it is situated where the still busy Fosse Way and the even busier Great North Road meet. This makes it something of a hazard to navigation if you are walking or using your on-board, folding cycle. It is no place at all for jay walking but is absolutely splendid for sight-seeing and shopping; that is, if you are not a martyr to impulse purchasing (or to others who are) for there is a plethora of antique shops, all with windows and contents that stare at you as if to defy you to walk past without proving for yourself that within their pricey artefacts or indeed their very denizens themselves they boast uniquely genuine proofs of Newark's longevity. There is something for almost every taste in this town, for it can boast the best and the worst from ancient and modern, especially to be noticed in its markets, market-place and shopping precincts. It is certainly a place of contrasts.

NEWARK
Cromwell Lock 5 miles
Nottingham 22 miles

Moorings
On both sides of the river below Town Lock there are BWB moorings. There are also a few just by the side of the new lock in the 'cut' that used to be the old lock.

Marina
Newark Marina Ltd., 26 Farndon Road, Newark. ☎ Newark (0636) 704022. (On the River Devon, pronounced Deev'n, with access for boats up to 5'. There is a full range of marine goods and services.)
Farndon Harbour, North End, Farndon, Newark NG24 3SX. ☎ Newark (0636) 705483. (Situated a couple of miles up river from Newark; in a pretty spot, with comprehensive facilities, goods and services.)

Boatyard
Facilities at the two marinas mentioned above.
Fiskerton Wharf, Fiskerton, Newark, Notts. NG25 0EP.
☎ Newark (0636) 830695.

Facilities

🚻 ⚓ ● ⛽ ✕ 🔧 ✉ 🏪 s 🚏

Remarks
Newark is well supplied with most of the normal (and many of the extraordinary) requirements of cruising folk. But there is no laundrette within laundry-bag-carrying distance.
Newark Marina is equipped with VHF radio: Call Sign *Newark Forecaster*. Channel 'M'.

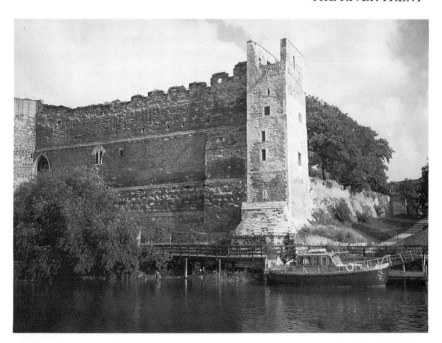

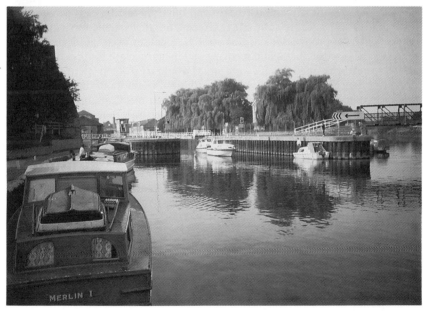

The Trent at Newark.

NEWARK NETHER LOCK

British Waterways Board
Nether Lock,
Newark,
Notts. NG24 2EE
☎ Newark (0636) 703830
VHF channels 16 and 74

Restricting dimensions - 190' x 30' x 7'8" (depth
of basin).
Rise and fall   depends on water levels
Mechanised   ●
Keeper operated   ●
Facilities nearby ⚓ ⬛

Remarks
See Cromwell Lock for operating times.

NEWARK TOWN LOCK

British Waterways Board
Newark Town Lock,
Castlegate,
Newark,
Notts. NG24 1BG
☎ Newark (0636) 702226
VHF channels 16 and 73

Restricting dimensions   190' x 30' x 8'9"*
Rise and fall   depends on water levels
Mechanised   ●
Keeper operated   ●
Facilities nearby
⚓ ⬛ ⌐S♪ ✉
🚶 in town

Remarks
*Limiting dimensions for navigation through
Newark relate to the channel and presence of
bends/bridges, etc. If in doubt – dimensions,
etc. of craft should be sent to the area office,
Nottingham who will advise whether craft can
navigate through Newark.
See Cromwell Lock for operating times.

Even if you have a boat of your own, I would still urge you to sample the
pleasures of a Trent trip on board *Sonning*, the truly terrific ex-Thames afternoon craft, run by Aubrey and Mary Green from their scenic mooring by the
castle. Their 'appropriation' of this stretch, together with the occupation of
much of the opposite bankside moorings by fishermen are sources of conster-
nation to local cruising folk. If I were you, I would try to keep out of any discus-
sion regarding the rights and wrongs of these dispensations; it seems something of a nine-day storm in a wonder-teacup. I last met Captain Aubrey when
I was iced up in Sheffield's Canal Basin, and I am happy to report that his present operation is even more attractive, well run and worthwhile than was the
Sheffield Water Bus Service. He has lost none of his smiling nonchalant charm
nor do the darts of his piercing insight into the human condition fly less often
or less accurately than they ever did. Make sure you enrol for a ride, ensuring
to sample the wares in the bar; and after the obligatory sip or two, engage him
in conversation and you will be in the running for two trips for the price of one.

Not far up river from Newark you will discover a succession of surprises; the
first is the size of the fantastic weir just before the equally fantastic power station near Farndon. They will be closely attended by a flock of geese that seem
to have taken over the river just after the next bend; and, intermingling with
them as if fully paid up members of that gaggle of ganders, can be seen, also
mixing and matching, representatives from many kinds of water birds from the
wheeling and dealing of the raucous young seagulls to the stilted and disdainful
erectness of the ageing herons. Just around the next bend from the concatena-
tion is another: a conglomerate of sailing, fishing, eating, drinking and any

other kind of relaxation that is usually associated with river and riverside life, all suitably symbolised by Farndon Harbour, the biggest marina on the Trent. It is headed and purposefully led by Mr. and Mrs. Ainsworth, an indubitable couple who are the co-operatively direct and directly co-operative directors. Set in the heart of the countryside, but with industry, commerce and business never far away, it must be one of the prettiest marinas in the country. It has everything you are likely to need, and is also the home of that veteran Trent Boating Association supporter, Sid Skegells and his *Trisha*, a South Ferriby (Clapson) built canoe-stern, motor-sailer.

Not far up river comes the village of Fiskerton (like its namesake near Lincoln, derived from its old nomenclature, *Fishers' Town*) and it is a spot that is worth going out of your way to visit, by road or by river. Here, you can hire a boat, eat at an Egon Ronay-type inn (although it may not strike you as being immediately appealing from the outside) and buy almost anything you are likely to need. If there ever was a cruising stop that I should wax lyrical about, it is Fiskerton. It has an excellent deep-water mooring by clean, well kept and substantial steps that lead almost directly to the Bromley Arms (the pub with the grub). A few yards distant, well camouflaged behind rustic brickery, but also well advertised by an emblazoned legend, is the home of Fiskerton Cruisers. The place was once a steam mill and maltings; now they moor craft and hire out narrow boats, and – somewhat surprisingly – they build, one at a time, ocean-going yachts. They also have a fuel and basic chandlery service. You will find them smilingly efficient and welcoming.

Just around the corner from the wharf is the village shop and post office; it is veritably stuffed with goodies that range from the necessaries to support life to all kinds of tasty, esoteric tit-bits. It is a real jewel in the crown of old-fashioned 'corner shops', and claims to be the only riverside shop between Newark and Nottingham. Their service is so enthusiastic that it even extends to publishing a small brochure about themselves: 'You can be guaranteed a friendly, personal service. If the village shop does not have what you want then you only have to ask for it . . . requests for even one egg or one slice of bacon are willingly provided.' Under the banner headline 'Save Money, Save Time, Save the Village: Use it or Lose it' the village shop at Fiskerton is campaigning away, and deserves a special visit from all passing skippers and their crews. If you like Torksey, you will find Fiskerton equally, but quite differently, appealing.

From Fiskerton onwards, up to Nottingham, there is a danger that this chapter will begin to sound like a catalogue of 'Best Stopping Places I have known on the River Trent'; and to a very real extent, visiting all the actual and potential stopping places is what cruising the upper reaches of the Trent is all about. Nevertheless, there are some locations that demand and deserve to be mentioned, and the first of these is Hazelford. The lock itself, although pleasant to look upon and with no navigational hazard, is not the subject of my enthusiasm; that is reserved for the lock-keeper – and anyone meeting him for the first time is in for an intriguing experience for he is an idiosyncratic fellow

HAZELFORD LOCK

British Waterways Board
Hazelford Lock,
Boat Lane,
Bleasby,
Nottingham NG14 7FT
☎ Newark (0636) 830312
VHF channels 16 and 74

Restricting dimensions 190' x 30' x 7'4"
Rise and fall depends on water levels
Hand operated ●
Keeper operated ●
Boater operated ●
Facilities nearby
⚓ ▱

Remarks
Hours of operation
Mon. 0800-1730
Tues.-Fri. 0700-1730
Sat. 0700-1200

GUNTHORPE LOCK

British Waterways Board
Gunthorpe Lock,
Trent Side,
Gunthorpe,
Notts. NG14 7FB
☎ Nottingham (0602) 663821
VHF channels 16 and 74

Restricting dimensions 190' x 30' x 9'
Rise and fall depends on water levels
Mechanised ●
Keeper operated ●
Facilities nearby

⚓ ᴡᴄ ▱ ♪ S

Remarks
See Cromwell Lock for operating times.

---

of 'infinite jest, of most excellent fancy'. His jest is just zest for life, and that is as it should be, but his excellent fancy is something else; it lies in his command of a vocabulary of hand, arm, face and body signals that gives an entirely new dimension to the concept of mime. Not only are his movements and gestures an aesthetic joy to behold merely on their own account (for they are wide ranging and well executed) but also, they are unmistakeably clear. Whether you are a novice or an expert, you will get the message straight away and without ambiguity: an advantage that will be recognised for its true worth by any skipper who has tried to understand what is being shouted at him from the lockside (or, perhaps worse, what is being relayed to him by those on board who think they understand) when all he can hear in the wheelhouse is the thunderous drumming of a pair of diesels not quite in sync. In any case, Hazelford is a welcoming spot and the pub is called the Star and Garter.

On then, past Hoveringham and another hostelry and small community, on to Gunthorpe; the enigma of the Trent. The village is a tourist trap without doubt, but it has still managed to retain some of the charm that it once must have had to have made it so popular now. However, that charm is difficult to discern and in the final resort must be described at best as residual or vestigial. That is, except for some notable exceptions: there is a totally unexpected mini-marina by the weir, looking absolutely picture-postcard pretty; there is also a small boatyard and marine service station (Damark Marine) where one of the Butlers is more than likely to take your ropes and assist you into a berth by the wall (where there is no shoaling close to); and, in addition, to serve other needs, there is the Yeoman Restaurant where they serve such delicacies as Ham Cornets filled with Cottage Cheese, Fisherman's Pot, Spatchcock Chicken, Pork Schnitzel and Sole Fourrées. Unlike some of those in this village apparently dedicated to serving the great British public, the folks at the Yeoman will spare you the time to do more than yawn in your face while they give you the bill. If Gunthorpe could be prised away from its devotion to Mammon, it would be a place to remember because of joyous, fresh experiences and not jaded, cynical exploitations.

Gunthorpe is biggish and busy, whereas the next port of call is smallish and busy; but busy in an entirely different kind of way. There are three things that bring folks flocking to Stoke Bardolph: the Ferry Boat Inn (with its dire warnings about what floods can do to people and buildings and what anti-flood boots can do to pub carpets); the favoured site for anglers; and the occasionally frenetic busy centre of it all, the sailing club. If there is space for you to moor up, you will find it a rewarding spot to spend a little time; and if you hanker after lots of socialising, then this must be a must.

The lock-keeper at Stoke Bardolph does all he can to help, but the paddles he has to work require so much brute force that your efforts will be welcome, and will speed on the process enormously. Boaters often 'help' lock-keepers when (a) there is no real need, and (b) when they would be better doing nothing for many get it wrong. But at this lock, a help in need is a help indeed. You will also find that some authorities still state that there is a ferry here (and in a number of other places as well) but you will be hard pressed to find those who even remember them plying for trade, never mind doing so now. Don't be misled into thinking that there is a marina by the weir; the boats are all moored at private berths quite near to the falling water.

The last outposts of rural river life before the spirit of Nottingham takes over are Holme Locks. There is one large and another small lock; boats with a draught exceeding 5′ should use the larger of the two, hoping that an improved system of mechanics will soon make it possible for one person to work the gates without being exhausted.

Then comes the quietly tucked away marina at Colwick Park, a spot that is miraculously still countryfied in spite of being so close to the city. It is worth noting that craft drawing much more than 1 metre will have to take very careful soundings on the way in. There is a red marker buoy to indicate the main shoal ground to be avoided (also the plenitude of weed) but there is not a lot of water around for a 6′ boat. Such craft can make use of the pontoons on the bank running along the outside of the marina, on the north side.

On the other side of the river (but with little to be seen from deck level) is the water sport centre at Holme Pierrepont, where they must be hoping that the Olympics will soon return to England. Nearer to Nottingham and on the other bank again comes the sophisticated estate of Merrill Brown Ltd., MB Park Marine and the Park Yacht Club, known to all as PYC. Here you can arrange for anything from a grand wedding reception to a grand gland packing; and from here, Trent Bridge and Nottingham proper will be in your sight.

Nottingham proper? Well, what could be more in keeping with the essence and spirit of Nottingham than a mooring by Trent Bridge, where nearby is to be found the Headquarters of the British Waterways Board Nottingham Area; the mooring, office and patrol vessel of the river police; Meadow Lane Lock,

STOKE LOCK

British Waterways Board
Stoke Lock,
Stoke Bardolph,
Notts. NG14 5HY
☎ Nottingham (0602) 878563
VHF channels 16 and 73

Restricting dimensions   190' x 30' x 9'6"
Rise and fall   depends on water levels
Hand operated   ●
Keeper operated   ●
Boater operated   ●
Facilities nearby
⚓
Remarks
See Hazelford Lock for operating times.

HOLME LOCK

British Waterways Board
Holme Lock,
Holme Pierrepont,
Nottingham NG2 2LU
☎ Nottingham (0602) 811197
VHF channels 16 and 73

Restricting dimensions   190' x 30' x 9'6"
Rise and fall   depends on water levels
Hand operated   ●
Keeper operated   ●
Boater operated   ●
Facilities nearby
⚓
Remarks
See Hazelford Lock for operating times. .

being the key to further inland waterways (in particular the River Soar and the Grand Union system); the famous cricket ground known all over the world as Trent Bridge; the equally famous (or should it be notorious?) football centre of Nottingham Forest; numerous huts, houses, clubs and clans all to do with river and riverside activities; and the imposing offices of the city council.

Meadow Lane Lock will prove to be the effective head of navigation if your craft exceeds the limiting dimensions of 81' x 14'6" x 3'6" x 8' air draught.

If you are unable to pass through this lock, there are moorings below Trent Bridge on the west bank and above it on the east bank by the council offices steps. (You should make sure that you steam at least 4-5 cables above the bridge before trying to cross to the steps or you will find shoal ground.) This second mooring could not be more pleasingly civilised, since it has all facilities to hand shoresides and an aspect that is attractively landscaped. The moorings are busy in season and the nearby roads are busy all the time.

The contrasts between the tidal and the non-tidal waters of the River Trent could hardly be more marked. The tidal stretches have few places where you can moor or anchor in complete comfort and safety without having crew on watch and it is best thought of as a river of passage, in particular providing access to the North Sea via the Humber or the Witham and Fossdyke. The non-tidal stretches, on the other hand, consist of one stopping place after another simply separated by a calm cruise that seldom lasts for longer than half an hour before the next possible staging post is in view. It is certainly not a stretch that calls for rigorous passage making; in fact, it is probably best appreciated if you look upon it as a series of round trips, on which you never actually go anywhere that can be called a cruise, but all of which offer something for everyone and tempt you to go back again and again. You can easily choose whether you want to be surrounded by nothing but trees (by a steeply wooded slope that denies access from the land) or to become part of a busy socialising set when you will never have a single lonely moment.

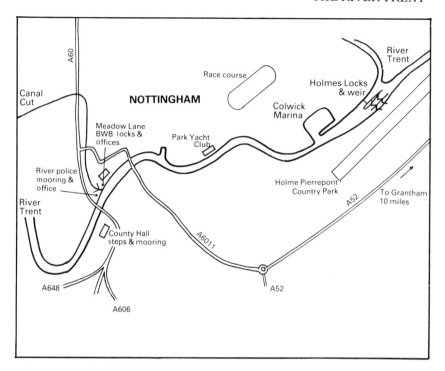

NOTTINGHAM
Cromwell Lock 27 miles

Moorings
Excellent moorings by the steps at County Hall. All domestic facilities are nearby.

Marina
M.B. Park Marine, The Old Pleasure Park, Trent Lane, Nottingham. ☎ Nottingham (0602) 506550. Comprehensive facilities.

Colwick Marina (just below Holme Locks) where there are a few visitors' moorings, but no domestic facilities nearby.

Boatyard
M.B. Park Marine are the people to contact.

Club
The Park Yacht Club at M.B. Park Marine.

Facilities

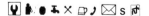

Remarks
One is more or less spoilt for choice of facilities, and provided you do not try to navigate far above County Hall, there is no hazard, other than the temptations of the trip to Jerusalem and the Goose Fair. The good deeds of Mr Boot do tend to dominate the city.

MEADOW LANE LOCK

British Waterways Board
Meadow Lane Lock,
Meadow Lane,
Nottingham
☎ (0602) 862414

Restricting dimensions 81' x 14'6" x 3' draught
Rise and fall depends on river levels
Hand operated •
Keeper operated • assistance at peak times
Boater operated •
Windlass required •

Facilities nearby

⚓ 🚾 🛗 S

🛢 at nearby garage

♪ ¼ mile

✉ ¼ mile

Remarks

The lock connects the River Trent to the Nottingham/Beeston Canal which is the route for navigation, through Nottingham rejoining the Trent at Beeston.

The River Trent is not available for through navigation between Meadow Lane Lock and Beeston, but craft may journey upstream of Meadow Lane Lock beyond Trent Bridge for about ¾ mile depending on draught of boat and river levels. There is good overnight mooring just upstream of Trent Bridge.

*Air draught is limited to approx. 7'9" by numerous bridges upstream of the lock.

Nottingham.

The locks also reflect the contrast: those in the tidal river can pose problems of access that are dictated by time and tide. 'Time and tide wait for no man'; but there is often a great deal of waiting by the lock-keepers on the non-tidal river if they happen to know that you are a bit late and rushing to meet a deadline of, if not exactly 'buttered eggs' (for they wait for no man either) then at least something quite important. Once upriver of Cromwell, you can carry on cruising within reason as and when you please. Similarly, the townships are also different: the hardiness and scant sophistication of places like Keadby and West Stockwith, coupled with the almost insurmountable problems of getting ashore from a cruiser in Gainsborough, are in tremendous contrast with the easily-in-reach cosmopolitan joys and contemporary entertainments that are patently and often blatantly on offer in Newark and Nottingham.

Once you know what you are doing in a boat that knows what it is doing (and is sea-kindly to boot) in the potentially fierce tidal waters, the 100 miles of the Trent will offer continuing change and splendid variety and, if you need one, a clean gateway to the sea, with no real hazard other than that of the British climate. The challenges of the next two waterways, which both run off the River Trent, are of an entirely different quantity and quality.

The River Idle

Once upon a time, the River Idle was free to come and go into the River Trent at West Stockwith at the dictates of the tides and weather. It was, of course, also free to flood the surrounding areas according to similar dictates and with the same lack of inhibition.

In 1935, the first sluice doors into the Trent became operable, and in 1981 a second set, with the addition of a powerful pumping station capable of pumping the Idle into the Trent even when the latter was higher than the former, also came into operation. Since then, pumping and sluicing have restrained the efforts of nature to flood the locality and the Idle no longer runs fast and free.

Local boat enthusiasts believe there is a serious possibility that they may be denied the navigation of the Idle in the future if they do not take steps to safeguard their rights.

However, I spoke with employees of the Severn/Trent Water Authority at three different levels in the hierarchy and all of them went out of their way to assure me that there was not, nor ever had been, any threat to the pleasure-and-leisure users of the Idle navigation. Two of the men most closely concerned with the sluicing operations at West Stockwith, Mr Woodcock and Mr Walker, carefully explained to me why it is not possible for boats to use the Idle without advance notification:

'Our main reasons for needing notice are twofold. We want to make sure that the pumps are turned off at the appropriate times, otherwise boats would in all probability be swamped; and we also want to make sure that the gates are open the correct amount otherwise boats will not be able to get through.'

What happens at other times is regulated automatically through sluicing, gateing and pumping operations that are controlled by sensors out in the River Trent at Owston Ferry. These sensors detect which way the river is flowing, and, dependent upon the difference in heights between the Idle and the Trent, open the gates and/or pump out into the Trent. The two gates in the Idle are about 300 yards apart and effectively create an enormous (and pleasingly turfed) lock that is quite without the snags of rushing water and protruding bolts, beams and masonry that bedevil many others. Since advance arrangements have to be made for entry into the Idle and any progress up the river may be affected by strongly local variations of tide, weather and freshwater levels,

DISTANCES

River Idle

	West Stockwith	Misterton Road Bridge	Idle Stop	Misson	Newington	Bawtry
West Stockwith		2	4	7	9	11
Misterton Road Bridge	2		2	5	7	9
Idle Stop	4	2		3	5	7
Misson	7	5	3		2	4
Newington	9	7	5	2		2
Bawtry	11	9	7	4	2	

Chesterfield Canal

	West Stockwith	Misterton	Gringley	Drakeholes	Clayworth	Hayton	Clayborough	Whitsunday Pie Lock	Retford	Ranby	Worksop
West Stockwith		2	4	6	9	11	13	14	15	20	25
Misterton	2		2	4	7	9	11	12	13	18	23
Gringley	4	2		2	5	7	9	10	11	16	21
Drakeholes	6	4	2		3	5	7	8	9	14	19
Clayworth	9	7	5	3		2	4	5	6	11	16
Hayton	11	9	7	5	2		2	3	4	9	14
Clayborough	13	11	9	7	4	2		1	2	7	12
Whitsunday Pie Lock	14	12	10	8	5	3	1		1	6	11
Retford	15	13	11	9	6	4	2	1		5	10
Ranby	20	18	16	14	11	9	7	6	5		5
Worksop	25	23	21	19	16	14	12	11	10	5	

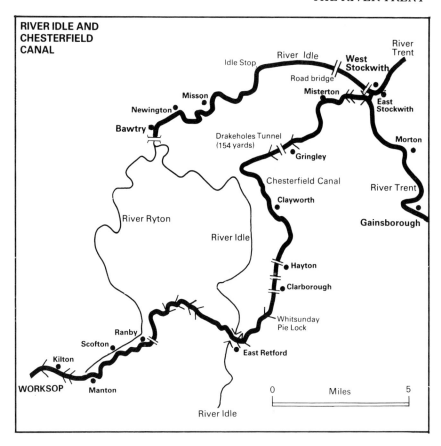

RIVER IDLE AND CHESTERFIELD CANAL

it must be best to lock into the Chesterfield Canal at West Stockwith (Lock No. 65) and stay over in the basin to check details with the keepers of the lock.

The Idle is a narrow river with fairly high banks. There is little to see along the eleven miles that proves civilisation to be near at hand: there is a pretty bridge by the Gate Inn; some attractive gardens running down to the river at Misson; an occasional glimpse of a road and a railway, a tractor and a sand quarry; and finally, a few people walking mainly with dogs just before Bawtry. Otherwise it is dandelions, docks and daisies all the way; and a few million weeds.

There are, of course, the obligatory 'private' notices that all riparian, territorially obsessed persons feel they must erect; but there are also, on a much happier note, many signs of the Severn/Trent Water Authority taking its responsibilities more than seriously in an area where it is only too easy to make excuses for doing nothing. They were not only completing the functional works on the bank in a very attractive manner, but also planting a plenitude of trees and grassing with grace and style.

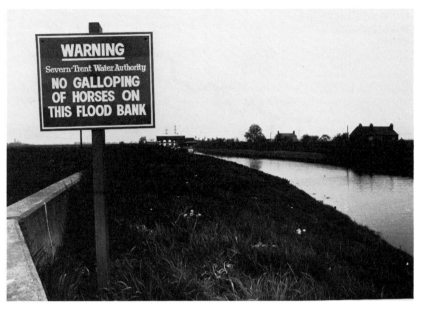

The grass-surrounded 'pound' on the River Idle looking upstream.

The amazingly large structure that controls the water on the amazingly unlarge waterway that is the River Idle .

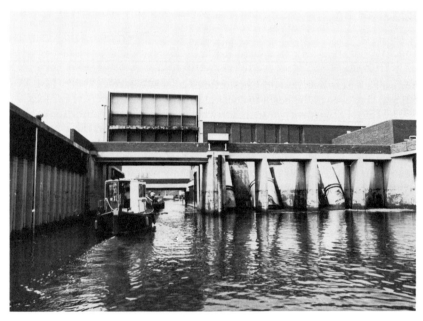

If you want to get away from it all, then the River Idle must be for you. On almost every day of the year (except the annual cruise of the Retford and Worksop Boat Club) there will be a 99% chance that you will not meet another craft. You may pass a fisherman, but you are likely to do that anywhere. Personally, I can see no threat that the river navigation will be closed, nor that the waters will become infested or even partly over-run by tourists. The only real danger must surely be that the charms of the Idle will inspire idylls that may lead to idolatry. There is an old proverb that runs: 'Of idleness comes no goodness'; but indeed to goodness there is plenty of it to be found on the Idle and in its fans . . . especially among the boating fraternity.

A similar kind of thing can be said of the Chesterfield Canal; another waterway with a fanatical fan club that will never let it become no more than a reminder of glories past, although it may well be, in fact, well and truly remaindered.

The Chesterfield Canal

The Chesterfield Canal is approached from the River Trent at West Stockwith Lock, and the basin gives onto the canal itself at its far end. The Trent tends to fall bleak and remote in this area, and the remoteness is continued once you are 'inland'. However, the bleakness begins to die away as something of the spirit of rural Nottinghamshire makes its presence felt. If you are looking for a waterway that has not been commercialised; is not packed with speedy hire boats or fast tourists even at the height of the season; nor is littered with floating pontoons at £5.00 a night and a disco at your door, then this canal will appeal to you.

There are sixteen locks in its 26 miles, and all but the one at West Stockwith for the River Trent are customer operated and while not all of them can be properly described as 'user friendly', generally speaking the stretch to Worksop is in good order. It is certainly a pretty cruise and there are plenty of interesting stopping places (especially if you are keen to watch unfettered and untroubled wildlife); but, like most of the non-commercial canals in the northeast, the channel is getting narrower and shallower season by season, so you must ensure that you have a decent plank if you are going to try to moor at any but the most used haunts.

The first village after West Stockwith is Misterton, hardly spitting distance away, and shortly after is Gringley-on-the-Hill. Both are worth exploring although you will have to walk about a mile and a half from the canal to get to the second, while the first offers immediate access. The next item to note is Drakeholes Tunnel which is quite straight, straightforward and runs for 154 yards. At its south end, there is a 90 degree bend which must be approached and navigated with caution; after which follow the two contrasted village communities of Wiseton and Clayworth – both, in their different styles, well worth exploring. Then comes what might be described as the *pièce de résistance* of the canal: the small market town of Retford. There are plenty of domestic facilities and the town is riddled with history, heritage and heritors who will be mightily

RETFORD

West Stockwith 15 miles
Worksop 10 miles

Moorings
In Retford Basin is to be found the Headquarters of the Retford Mariners Boat Club and there are some 'grace and favour' moorings with them – with prior permission. There are moorings both below and above Town Lock.

Boatyard
The nearest is at West Stockwith.

Club
The Retford Mariners Boat Club is in the Canal Basin. ☎ Retford (0777) 702705
The Retford and Worksop Boat Club is at Clayworth Wharf. ☎ Retford (0777) 817546.

Facilities
🏃 ● ⚓ ✕ 🕯 �bar/S

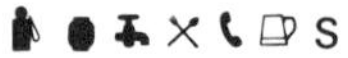

Remarks
There is a 70' turning place near Gas House Bridge and another near Woodcock's Bridge.
Do try to talk them into giving you afternoon tea at the White Hart Hotel in the market place.

WORKSOP

West Stockwith 26 miles

Moorings
Suitable moorings giving easy access to the town and its full range of domestic facilities.
There is a BWB maintenance yard alongside the canal: ☎ Worksop (0909) 472788.
The nearest marina and boatyard are at West Stockwith.

Remarks
Worksop is a dream of a place (just ponder over the Old Ship Inn!) that is, and probably always was, an anachronism; for there can be little doubt that what it stands for today has never really had a pure existence at any time in its history – and its commercial future sits uneasily upon the back of its much vaunted heritage. Altogether a fascinating place.

pleased to tell you at length precisely what it is about what they have inherited that they so jealously guard – and in particular will lead you a merry dance if you want more than superficial information about the amazingly named Whitsunday Pie Lock.

Next comes a series of memorable names: Ranby, Scofton, Osberton (Hall and Park), Worksop and, finally, but sadly beyond the head of navigation that is to be found at Morse Lock on the further outskirts of Worksop, the quaintly named Rhodesia. There are facilities for domestic needs at all of these ports of call, with the biggest and best being Worksop.

I vividly remember being taken to both Retford and Worksop as a child to enjoy the Sunday afternoon delights that were supposed to be offered by the Dukeries, especially the fact and mythology of Sherwood Forest. Cream teas were the usual bribe for afternoons of totally boring and quite misleading pseudo-history.

For those readers who are possessed of boats suitable to navigate to the very last rod, pole or perch of this charming waterway, I would recommend *The Chesterfield Canal*, which goes into comprehensive detail about the canal with all the references needed for full enjoyment by boaters, walkers, cyclists or four-wheel tourists. It is published by the Chesterfield Canal Society (for details, please refer to the recommended reading list).

III. THE SHEFFIELD & SOUTH YORKSHIRE NAVIGATION

The Stainforth & Keadby Canal

I have written elsewhere about Keadby (the River Trent: pp.71-8) but there is always a little bit more to be said about this place that is so idiosyncratic and incorrigible in its indigenes and the company it keeps. To this day, I can remember my first visit by water to Keadby. (Long before then, Keadby had been known to my schooldays *copins* as a refuge for our under-age smoking and drinking – and general coming to terms with adolescent struggles for dominance in a world that seemed to dominate us somewhat cruel.) There were what I now know to be the usual mud spits; a couple of coasters – one at each jetty; little enough water anyway for I was navigating on what was, for me, the last of the ebb; and a series of unpleasant swirls and whirls at the entrance, caused by the configuration of the ships and jetties . . . and aided and abetted by one of the coasters churning away with its stern propeller. All in all, I had a rough, tough time of it, and in the end had to get *Valcon* into the entrance astern, since that was the only way she would allow herself to be handled in the depth that she was floating in. When I finally got a line ashore, having passed through those massive wooden gates that guard Keadby against flooding, I was greeted by the keeper of the keys: 'I've locked more boats in and out of here than you've had hot dinners; but I've never seen one come in that way before. What do you think you are, a crab with wings?'

Thus spake the Zarathustra of the lock; with great condescension, little patience and absolutely no sympathy for me, the licence-holding navigator who had struggled to quit the Trent for the calmer, non-tidal waters of the Stainforth & Keadby Canal. It was neither the most exciting nor the most soothing of welcomes; but it did at least sort-of-guarantee that things would get better; after all, they could hardly get worse? And get better they did; that keeper and I are still not yet 'buddies', but we are almost comrades – and I have come to respect the hard graft that the keepers must employ to operate the system at Keadby, and to understand why they are always on the *qui vive* for those eccentricities of boat handling that so frequently come their way . . . and usually mean trouble. (On the other hand, it must also be said that there are all sorts in lock-keepers as there are in life; and one or two of them seem psychologically made up in a manner that actually prevents them from being either cheerful or courteous. I have seen some of them going through the hoops as they do the very best they can be to be polite and friendly; and I have seen them struggle, and fail.)

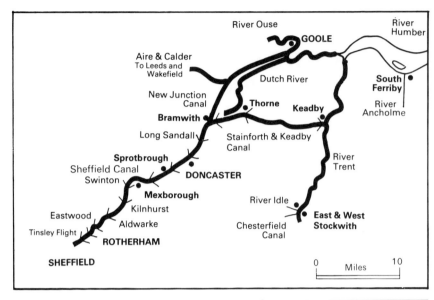

SHEFFIELD & SOUTH YORKSHIRE NAVIGATION

Keadby to Bramwith Junction 14 miles. (Stainforth & Keadby Canal)

Bramwith Junction to Aire & Calder Junction 5 miles. (New Junction Canal)

Bramwith Junction to Sheffield Canal Basin 28 miles. (Sheffield Canal)

Non-tidal throughout.

Dimensions
Length 60'
Beam 15'
Draught 6' (but see text)
Air draught 10' (but see text)

Locks
Stainforth & Keadby 3
New Junction 1
Sheffield 24

Traffic
There is little traffic of any kind from Rotherham to Sheffield; the only traffic on the Stainforth & Keadby for some time has been light pleasure craft in the main, with one working barge; but the rest of the waterway plays host to barges and Tom Puddings of substance.

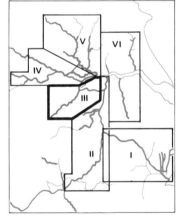

Remarks
Some parts of the waterway (especially the Stainforth & Keadby and even more so the run from Rotherham to Sheffield) are used so little that they are tending to silt up in certain stretches and the limit of 6' is an absolute maximum for craft at dead slow speed; and the air draught of 10' is only possible in comfort if the craft is not of the full beam at that height.

OS Maps (1:50,000)
112 Scunthorpe
111 Doncaster

TABLE OF DISTANCES

	Keadby	Crowle	Thorne	Stainforth	Bramwith	Sykehouse	Aire and Calder Junction	Barnby Dun	Doncaster	Sprotbrough	Mexborough	Swinton	Rotherham	Tinsley Flight	Sheffield Canal Basin
Keadby		3	10	12	14	17	19	16	21	24	29	31	36	39	42
Crowle	3		7	9	11	14	16	13	18	21	26	28	33	36	39
Thorne	10	7		2	4	7	9	6	11	14	19	21	26	29	32
Stainforth	12	9	2		2	5	7	4	9	12	17	19	24	27	30
Bramwith	14	11	4	2		3	5	2	7	10	15	17	22	25	28
Sykehouse	17	14	7	5	3		2	5	10	13	18	20	25	28	31
Aire & Calder Junction	19	16	9	7	5	2		7	12	15	20	22	27	30	33
Barnby Dun	16	13	6	4	2	5	7		5	8	13	15	20	23	26
Doncaster	21	18	11	9	7	10	12	5		3	8	10	15	18	21
Sprotbrough	24	21	14	12	10	13	15	8	3		5	7	12	15	18
Mexborough	29	26	19	17	15	18	20	13	8	5		2	7	10	13
Swinton	31	28	21	19	17	20	22	15	10	7	2		5	8	11
Rotherham	36	33	26	24	22	25	27	20	15	12	7	5		3	6
Tinsley Flight	39	36	29	27	25	28	30	23	18	15	10	8	3		3
Sheffield Canal Basin	42	39	32	30	28	31	33	26	21	18	13	11	6	3	

Navigation authority
British Waterways Board,
Castleford Area,
Lock Lane,
Castleford WF10 2LH
☎ (0977) 554351/5
After hours 554351 connects with Securicor
Bradford for emergency use.

Water authority
Yorkshire Water,
21 Park Square South,
Leeds LS1 2QG
☎ (0532) 440191

It was at Keadby, that I was introduced to Jean Ingelow's poem, *High Tide on the Coast of Lincolnshire*. In it she refers to something like the Trent bore (that great tidal wave with a precipitous front), the word 'bore' coming from the Old Norse *bara* and meaning a wave or billow. It is, of course, also known by other names equally old and equally threatening; for example, the Severn and Trent Water Authority refer to it as an aegir (and that is also Old Norse, meaning God of the Sea), while many Lincolnshire experts insist that it is an eagre or eager (being, in its turn, Old English for 'flood'). Jean Ingelow's poem does nothing to clarify the spelling:

'A mighty eygre reared his crest,
And uppe the Lindis raging sped.
It swept with thunderous noises loud;
Shaped like a curling snow-white cloud,
Or like a demon in a shroud.'

KEADBY See also text pages 75-6

Trent Falls 10 miles
West Stockwith 12 miles
Cromwell Lock 43 miles
Thorne 10 miles

Moorings
There are two main jetties outside the lock: one immediately downstream of the entrance and one above it. The one above it is sometimes available to pleasure craft; and even if occupied, it may be that the commercial skipper will be co-operative and take your lines. Downstream of the entrance is to be avoided by all pleasure craft; and upstream you should notify the lock-keeper of your presence, just in case he hasn't seen you arrive! Inside the lock (after the huge doors and the road swing bridge) there are moorings on each side of the canal. In season, they tend to be very crowded, and often there are queues alongside the water and sanitary station – sometimes rafted up.

Facilities nearby

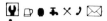

🐾 Only in the village
S (must be described as 'limited')

Remarks
The entrance to the lock can be complicated by the rate of flow of the flood; the two mud spits that strike out from the entrance knuckles; and the presence of a number of coasters, sometimes making sight lines and the approach run tricky . . . especially if they happen to have their screws turning as they are known to do.

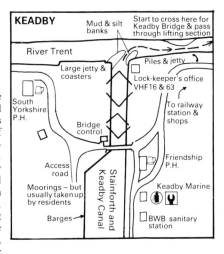

KEADBY LOCK

BWB Keadby Lock,
Trentside,
Keadby,
Scunthorpe
North Humberside
☎ Scunthorpe (0724) 782205
VHF channels 16 and 74

Restricting dimensions   77'8" x 21'10"
Rise and fall   tidal
Hand operated   ●
Keeper operated   ●

Facilities nearby

⚓ 🚻 📕

🛥 Keadby Marine Ltd. above lock
  ☎ (0724) 782302
📳 Friendship ☎ (0724) 782243
S General stores
✉ 2 minutes walk
🔧 200 yards from lock
⚓

Remarks
At this tidal lock please notify the lock-keeper of your estimated time of arrival giving 24 hours notice if possible.

Opening times:
Monday-Thursday 0600-2200 hours
Friday 0600-2000 hours
Saturday 0700-1200 hours
          1300-1700 hours
Sunday 0900-1200 hours
        1300-1700 hours
Short term shelter passes for unlicensed and unregistered craft available at this location. Current details from the lock-keeper.

However, there is no ambiguity about what she is describing. No wonder I used, as a child, to think of that eagre as some Neptunian ogre and could never understand why bus, transport and construction companies were named after it.

Back on the canal, though, any conflicts of that scale are always man made; the waters themselves are troubled only by a lack of depth, care and protection not having been used extensively for many years. After its construction around the turn of the 18th century, the Stainforth & Keadby actually flourished dramatically for 150 years and was an important lifeline in the area's industry and commerce. But ever since 1960 it has become less and less significant and it is now, in the main, a reservation for fishermen and boating enthusiasts. Sadly, these two groups, which are generally almost mutually exclusive, usually become involved with one another only in getting their lines entangled and in no way seem to set out to try to make life and leisure harmonious for one another. Nevertheless, they are united in their hopes that British Waterways will keep the canal in a decent state of preservation.

The first attempts to make the nearby River Don navigable right up to the satanic mills and hills of Rotherham and Sheffield were made as long ago as 1697, but it was not until 1751 that boats actually got as far as Tinsley. Fifty years later, a canal was constructed from Stainforth to the River Trent with entrance locks at Thorne and Keadby. (The remains of the construction at Stainforth can still be seen where Stanilands retain a small mooring station.) In 1815, a horse passenger packet started to run between Thorne and Keadby and continued until about 1840. But it was not until 1895 (about 100 years after the rest of the country had experienced its canal mania) that the diminutive waterway now known as the Stainforth & Keadby line became an integral part of the Sheffield & South Yorkshire Navigation, thus affording the latter a new port and outlet at Keadby. Ironically enough, it was only 10 years later that the New Junction was opened, creating straightforward competition with its port and outlet at Goole. In spite of its fall from grace and favour and its continued parlous state in many stretches, it is nevertheless not a waterway to be ignored – and it all starts at Keadby.

By any standards Keadby is an intriguing place; being a something-and-nothing community where everyone will talk to you, but few will say very much. On the surface, little or nothing at all is going on, but once any superficial judgment has been suspended in favour of a deeper enquiry, it soon becomes clear that matters of great pith and moment are being debated, and deeds of great import and significance being executed. While the general air may be one of deprivation, poverty and depression, upon close observation and singular encounters, one is forced to the conclusion that there is nary a soul who is not buoyant now or optimistic for later. They may not be all at one with life, but they are certainly not at sixes or sevens with it. The lock and swing bridge may be as cumbersome and threatening as any ancient engine of war, and the muddied swirling waters at the entrance may command great respect but hold little appeal; but nevertheless the rest of the village, from the most southerly point of extremely general stores and railway bridge to the stern outlook of the seafaring *hombre* who positively glares down from the Sign of the Mariners, is an experience to relish, and not, as many travellers must these days, one to ignore or lightly pass by. In fact most people do give Keadby a miss, and they are wrong; for it is packed with interest (shops may indeed be few, but every keeper is a phenomenon to relish) and redolent of those days now gone by when industrial and commercial architecture was of a quality to catch the eye of every passing Dante Gabriel Rossetti.

VAZON SWING BRIDGE

Keadby,
Scunthorpe,
South Humberside
VHF channels 16 and 74

Restricting dimensions   22′ wide bank to bank
Hand operated   •
Keeper operated   •
Facilities nearby None

Remarks
Opening times:
Monday-Thursday 0800-1200 hours
                              1230-1630 hours
Friday 0800-1200 hours
            1230-1530 hours
Saturday 0800-1200 hours
                1300-1700 hours
Sunday 0900-1200 hours
              1300-1700 hours

GODKNOW SWING BRIDGE

Crowle,
Scunthorpe,
South Humberside

Restricting dimensions   22′ bank to bank.
Hand operated   •
Keeper operated   •
Facilities nearby None

Remarks
See Vazon Swing Bridge for opening times.

MEDGE HALL SWING BRIDGE

Crowle,
Scunthorpe,
South Humberside

Restricting dimensions   22′ bank to bank.
Hand operated   •
Keeper operated   •
Facilities nearby None

Remarks
See Vazon Swing Bridge for opening times.

And so are the works that you will next encounter along the canal route just past the power station: a rail bridge, all metal, known to stick quite often and with little effort or to suffer from power failure; and a road bridge, mainly wood, known to require much effort before it can be coaxed into budging – but fortunately looked after by a single-handed, single-minded keeper who himself, thankfully, does not suffer from any kind of power failure. Should you need to wait upon the vagaries of either of these bridges, there is a good mooring by the wall on the starboard hand before the railway and another immediately inside the small pond or pound that separates the two bridges. This is on the port hand; the rest of the pond is fairly shallow at the banks and the facilities for tying up are not good. Both bridge-keepers respond happily to sound signals.

After these two aspects of 'power', there is a small collection of boats on the starboard hand, and you may well see one or two of the Sea Scouts MFV conversions around there. After this, there is little of interest until you reach Crowle, where broken down buildings and a nasty wharf offer a reminder of how pathetic we have been in letting our waterways and their waterside communities become derelict. On both sides there are buildings just waiting for decent treatment and the whole place could become a joy to look at and a much needed amenity. Crowle itself is a good mile away, with the nearest small community being Ealand.

After the motorway bridge it is not long before you will encounter the next of the hand-operated bridges for which this stretch of waterway is famous. This one is known as Godknow Bridge and it is followed a mile later by Crook o' Moor (known by most people as Medge Hall bridge, for there is a farm of that ilk close by; indeed, I remember it well from the 1939-45 war when part of my school 'war effort' was to work on that very farm – and it was there that I was introduced to the joys of cold tea (without milk or sugar) as a refreshment that could not be bettered in the heat of the day after a sweating stint that had started at 0500). Then comes a long straight stretch, accompanied on the north bank by the railway line and on the south by South Soak and Old Godknow Drains. Maud's Bridge is followed by Moor's Bridge, both hand-operated by keepers, and the last bridge to open before Thorne is reached is one of the new mechanised bascule bridges. Along this stretch there is every chance that you will be greeted by two or three horse/ponies that always appear to have seen better days and even the donkey that often walks (I was going to say 'runs' but that it not quite what it does) with them wears an unhappy mask. After this, it will not be long before you reach the outskirts of Thorne and the new development started by Tom Glen: Blue Water Marina.

It must be said that Blue Water is something of a euphemism for the appearance of the Adam's Ale that Tom let in in the spring of 1982, but for a symbol of what he is trying to achieve it is by no means a misnomer. The pool is 500′ x 120′ x 9′ and can accept craft with the maximum dimensions to get through Thorne lock: 60′ x 14′ x 5′6″. The entrance to the pool from the canal is 22′ wide, which is the same as the width of Keadby Lock. On completion, there will be 120 berths.

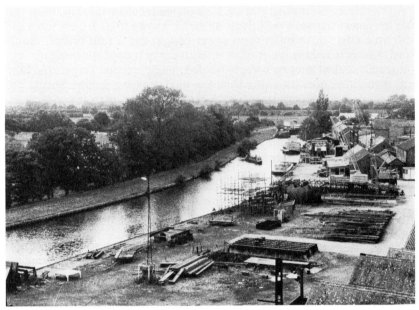

The Stainforth & Keadby Canal at Thorne looking up to the lock with Dunstan's shipyard on the right .

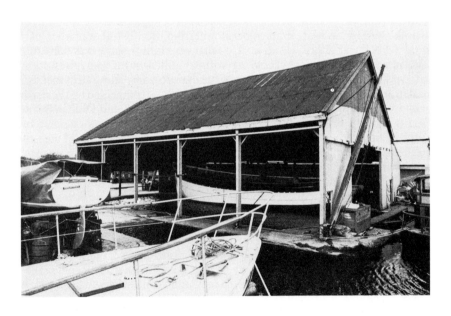

Staniland's covered dry dock, where much traditional work goes on.

THORNE

Keadby (for the Trent) 10 miles
New Junction Canal 5 miles

Moorings
Thorne possesses plenty of moorings – all over the place. BWB in the centre; Blue Water Marina at South End; Stanilands above the lock; Ladyline below the 'new' road bridge; and many other 'open' sites.

Marina
Blue Water Marina, South End. ☎ Thorne (0405) 813165.
Stanilands Boatyard, Lock Lane. ☎ Thorne (0405) 813150.

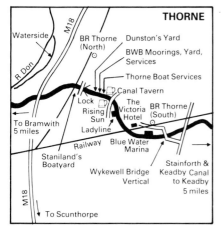

Boatyard
Stanilands, Lock Lane
Dunstons, Canalside
Blue Water Marina
Thorne Boat Services, South End,
☎ Thorne (0405) 814197

Club
Stanilands Clubhouse, The Boatyard
Thorne Boat Club, Blue Water Marina (Victoria Inn)

Facilities

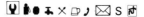

MAUD'S SWING BRIDGE *
MOORS SWING BRIDGE *
WIKEWELL BRIDGE *

*Address, dimensions, facilities and operation as for Medge Hall Swing Bridge. Opening hours as for Vazon Swing Bridge.

THORNE LOCK

Lock House,
Thorne,
Doncaster,
South Yorkshire
☎ (0405) 813110

Restricting dimensions 61'6" x 17'6"
Rise and fall 7'
Hand operated •
Keeper operated •
Facilities nearby
🚶 wc

🔧 Available at Marinas
🚶 (Petrol in town and near Blue Water Marina)
🛒 1 mile to town centre – several pubs
S 1 mile to town centre. Everything required.
♪ 1 mile
⚓ Stanilands, Blue Water Marina, BWB office

Remarks
See Vazon Swing Bridge for opening times.

Tom started the venture, in what was an old orchard with a couple of BWB cottages on it, as a result of 20 years 'old hankering and yearning'. His passion started in Port Harcourt, Nigeria and was consolidated later when he was the mooring officer at Apapa, the Port of Lagos. He worked on the trains of houseboats that moved about in 'colonies' of about 20: 'Drop anchor and drill here; there could be oil!' He is working up to a marina that will have a small chandlery, a clubhouse and an engineering repair station. There will be water, electricity and a station on the canal bank. Tom is offering a good service and deserves to succeed. He himself puts what he is trying to do this way: 'We set out to provide boat owners with what we know we have always looked for in boatyards and marinas ourselves.'

Nearby, there is an excellent engineer who will turn out at all kinds of unseemly hours and go to almost unseemly lengths to help you sort out your problem without it costing you an arm and a leg. Mr. Guest is a man to know about; though when you call on him, you may find him looking more like a farmer than an engineer – and your ears may be deafened by some of the noisiest dogs in the neighbourhood . . . but always in the way of welcoming you once they have established your good intentions.

According to the Ordnance Survey map (1:25,000 sheet SE 61/71 Thorne) South End is known as Wike Well End; but in a place where there are not only many names for almost every single street but also many houses with more than one number, this cannot be rated as really unlikely. For example, around Ellison Street towards South End you will find the dwellings numbered as follows: 7a (I could find no number smaller, so this must be the beginning) 9, 9a, 11, *Shangri La*, 13, 15, 19, and then quite normally from 21 to 29, but then another gap to 35, then 45, and, not to be outdone at the very end was a single house with the two numbers 49 and 51. After that, there is a pub, The Victoria, and no doubt many a frustrated visitor calls there in desperation.

Thorne is an intriguing spot; a small market town of contrasts, the biggest of which is that while any socio-economic survey would declare it dead and dodo-esque, it will neither lie down or be trampled underfoot; although it must be said that it is symbolically from its knees that it Dadaistically pursues its own tail, pausing only occasionally to take note (including those that fold) of what the rest of the world might be doing. Razor sharp, albeit low level, commerce flourishes in Thorne, and it has been said of its market place: 'The fast buck stops here.'

The very first thing that ever caught my eyes about Thorne was a street poster advertising the performance by some local thespians of *Love on the Dole*. Somehow, that brand new, blue and white poster, together with its legend, seemed to sum up the *genius loci*. But, when asking a market trader about this and that, he took my arm in a vice-like grip and said: 'I can sell anything here, so long as it isn't blue. I don't know why. The Thorne lot won't have anything at all to do with blue; yet they are the narrowest-minded Conservatives I come across on my circuit.'

Certainly Thorne is a collection of oddities and contradictions, and they abound everywhere: the town council calls it a market town and nearby Moorends a village; but I found little justification for either description and how the two can ever have been looked on as a single entity I cannot imagine. In this case, it is not a question of east is east and west is west, but rather one of north is north and south is south . . . and then there is Moorends. The reason being that Thorne has had two railway stations ever since 1860 or so; but the two sets of lines connect as little as do Thorne itself and its satellite Moorends. Both stations are on the outskirts and never do the twain trains meet, but it makes no difference at which one you alight, there will still be the same kind of buildings; all of great character but owing little to art, architecture, achievement or aesthetics – and from the vantage point of the water tower (contemporary concrete brutish) it is difficult to perceive why the centre of Thorne was declared a conservation area under the terms of the Civic Amenities Act.

Conservationists will not be pleased by the constant noise created by rolling stock; it is a pollution that can be heard all over Thorne, and it continues day and night although not uninterrupted. Nor for that matter is the sound of whirring and whining from model aeroplanes particularly pleasant, and it is usually encountered throughout weekends especially early on Sunday mornings when you are moored by the BWB offices and yard by the 'new' bridge. On the credit side however, it must be noted that in the area of Blue Water Marina you will be able regularly to hear the much more satisfactory sounds of frogs at play (or what you will); and, when all else is quiet and still, the delightful songs from the few larks that foregather around the basin.

Thorne is built on a ridge of sand about two miles long, and most of the area is little more than 5′ above sea level and none of it more than 25′. Its name derives from the Saxon: 'the place where the thorns grow'. It is variously spelled 'Torn', 'Thurne', 'Tourne' and 'Thourne'; so, in an area where boats are referred to as 'booerts' it can come as no surprise to meet locals who talk about 'Thooern'. Although the accents and dialects used in these parts are perfectly pure northeast Midlands (whatever that may be) your chances of hearing an actual pure vowel in the locality are very remote.

Its history lies deep in the past, about 10,000 years past. Later were the Romans (A.D. 50) who came to much grief at the hands of the local Brigantes. They were followed by the Saxons, the Christians, the Vikings and, in 1609, one Cornelius Vermuyden who was to revolutionise life in the east and whose much celebrated drainage schemes did not always work as well as they might have done: 1681: 'A great flood with high winds did break our banks in several places and drowned our towne around on Sunday night.'

Just to the north of Thorne and immediately next the River Don lies the old Thorne Quay now known as Waterside. It was the river port of Thorne from the early 18th century, having prospered after the floods that swept away the staith of the Dutch 'New Cut.' Brindley recommended a canal in 1763 and the navigation was opened in 1802 with a lock at Keadby for ships of up to 200 tons. Thorne is still redolent of the past and not least in its relic of a lock, complete with the far-too-close-for-comfort diminutive swing bridge that still works, apparently defying the laws of science, in spite of its image and muddy vestures of decay – but not, let it be emphasised, without the refuge and strength, the very present help in or out of trouble, of Mel, the long-suffering, indefatigable keeper of the bridge and its attendant gates.

Also closely attached to the past and illuminating stories of what life was really like, was a lady I met back at the quay, as it were, in her cottage at Waterside. She was a lithe and lively woman of mature years, a Mrs. Evelyn Holt, whose tales of canal and keel life were all informed with a spirit of sweetness and light without a single trace of mud or decay. Her enthusiasm could not have been keener if she had had canals instead of arteries, and she was good enough to tell me many a tale:

'My parents, William Guest Patrick and Maria Graham, were married in 1888; Dad was 21 and Mum 18. Afterwards, they went straight to Dad's keel, the *Hannah & Harriet* in Waddington's yard at Mexborough. Mum's first trip was her honeymoon taking coal from Denaby to Hull. Dad and a mate called Old Tom hauled from Mexborough, taking turns to pull, then to steer on board while eating the meal that Mum had got ready; her not being able to steer or anything. Then it was on to Doncaster for a Horse Marine to haul to Keadby, picking up their masts and leeboards at Thorne.

Dad said he would tow from Keadby to Hull on account of the honeymoon, and not sail as he usually did. Dad did most of the steering with Mother sat in the hatchway, her eyes like saucers at the buoys and sandbanks. In Hull the tug would turn round with the keels to face the ebb and drift them into place. This one day, a fishing trawler got caught by the ebb and rammed the line. Dad was last and so got the worst of it and Mother went right over the side. She went under the stern and under the coggy and was only kept up by the air pocket in her blouse. Dad, Old Tom and the keelmen got her out at last. She was unconscious and had to have treatment and was bad for two days. She was alright in the end; but what a honeymoon!

I was mate with Dad for 18 years and all the lightermen, dockers and keelmen would call me 'matey'. Once when we were loading locust beans, one of the dockers called me over to another boat and threw me down so many hands of green bananas that they nearly sank the coggy; but I was popular when we got back to Thorne! Often the kids would ask for bungy, a kind of sugary sweet stuff from the locust beans, and when I would say we had none, they would reply, 'Oh yes you have; we could smell it all the way from Goole.'

Sometimes, if we got caught against the tide, Dad would put me ashore with a line and seal: a belt 6" wide made of canvas or sail cloth that fits around the chest and shoulders and is attached to a line to the barge. I had to pull the keel as hard as I could, throwing the line over the willows and then dodging the branches. Dad would be pushing with the boat hook and steering at the same time. One farmer called out to his wife: 'Tha'd best bring thow'd gray mare from't stables an' tether her to this poor lass pulling this booert.' And if we didn't have briggage and the cargo was needed urgently we would have to take a line ashore and fasten it securely to a tree and then wind to the other with a sheet roller. Heaving like this was a slow job, as you had to take one line along at a time while the other held the boat. You can imagine I was pleased this did not happen very often.'

After the accident with the keel *Hannah & Harriet*, it was taken to Staniland's yard, and today Evelyn's husband Edgar works relief shifts there at the weekends. This yard is also a place of the past and the present: in their covered shed in the winter of 1983 was *Majessa*, a pleasure cruiser laid down in 1939 and finished in 1945, and nearby on the moorings was a 60' twin-screw motor boat laid down in 1934, *Bianda*, both having returned to their birth-yard after many years; and all around were the expensive, sleek lines of many GRP cruisers, some redolent of a real Italian Job.

The yard was opened by one John Staniland at Thorne Quay (now Waterside) in 1842. In 1863, his son was apprenticed and in 1869 they launched an 84 ton schooner, the *Black Cat* (84' x 20' x 10'6") which went missing at sea in 1923. In 1899, Isaac Margreave started at 14 years of age; in 1920, George Hunt Staniland, Mr. Margreave and a Mr. Naylor owned the yard. Mr. Staniland died, Mr. Naylor retired and Ron Margreave, the present owner, started his apprenticeship and gained full control in 1965. The last 'Sheffield size' barge was built in 1922 of massive timbers: 2" English oak planks with a breast of 18" x 12". When they had to put ¾" bolts in, it used to take a day to get the auger through. All the planks were steamed at the yard, and when I innocently but no doubt naïvely asked when was the last time that that operation had been carried out at the yard, Ron smiled quietly and said, 'Last week.'

Then along came a certain Captain Hylands of Wakefield who started to factor wooden motor cruisers; and in 1922 the first 36' boat was put down in a little wooden shed that had been an army hut. Ron's father was in charge at that time, and had never seen a plan in his life. Over 200 examples of the Hylands co-operation were built. At the same time they continued with barge repairs and conversions to diesel, and it was not until 1960-70 that barge work fell away completely. During the war the yard built 25' naval pinnaces, 24' RAF runabouts and 40' seaplane tenders. The contracts used to come in at about 12 a time, and all in all Stanilands built more than 100. Their largest pleasure cruiser was 68' x 18' and built in a shed that was no more than 70' x 20'. She was all teak, including the hull. In 1934, a twin-screw motor cruiser at 36' x 9' would have cost £1,200, and the last one they built was a 30' Zulu in 1970 at a cost of £6,000.

Now Ron takes what work there is: from lifeboat repairs to chandlery, engineering, general repairs, and the marina business. As he says: "Life brings its own patterns. If Life says, 'build boats'; you build 'em. If it says 'repair boats'; you repair 'em. Store 'em; paint 'em; whatever Life says, that's what you get on with." There is a thriving community here and it is well worth a visit. Ron Margreave himself is a man of not many words; but those you manage to coax from him will always be rewarding.

Next comes the lock and antiquated bridge, followed by Dunstons' Yard where in 1858 Richard Dunston began to build barges. In no time at all his yard was also making sails, ropes and running gear, and supplying all kinds of materials and equipment to the local trade, and also to the chandlers at Hull and Grimsby. Towards the end of the 19th century, they were standardising on

Sheffield keels and Humber sloops. Around 1920, sweeping changes brought plans for iron and steel ships and tugs of up to 700 b.h.p. and 300 d.w.t. coasters and lighters. Over the years, the great majority of tugs ordered for the River Thames have come from this yard, and while the recession of the early 1980s did not leave them unscathed, they are still in business and still optimistic.

(While researching something entirely different, in Hiscock's *Cruising under Sail* I came across the following: ' . . . the Hon. R. A. Balfour, now Lord Riverdale, produced the first of his line of Bluebirds in 1923. The year he was elected Commodore of the Royal Cruising Club, in collaboration with Arthur Robb, he designed the 21 ton yawl, Bluebird of Thorne. She was of twin keel design and was built of steel by Richard Dunston Ltd. in 1963.)

Close by Dunstons' are the yard and offices of the British Waterways Board. There is also a potentially very pretty mooring spot, but it is restricted to boats of very shallow draught; however, there is a length of quayside that is available for overnight stays close by.

And close by again is the well organised Thorne Boat Services, where you can get fuel, comprehensive chandlery and spares, and, above all, a unique kind of efficient service: you will not find a red carpet running down to the fuel point, nor a crowd of white-overalled palefaces to over-awe you while doffing their caps and assessing your bank balance; indeed, your introduction might well be the fiery barking of the guard dog, but after that what you will find is a keen working family unit led by Stuart Simpson. He is bright eyed, bushy bearded and will often intrigue you with brilliant asides that go to illuminate some of his enigmatic views on life. When it comes to boats and their insides however, there is nothing at all unusual about him except his expertise and general helpfulness: he will have a go at most things, and has established something of a corner in outboards in the area. You couldn't be in better hands.

Next comes the 'new' road bridge, and if you can manage to resist the wiling ways of the two nicely contrasted hostelries you will find a kind of new-and-second-hand emporium run by Ladyline. It is not the smoothest nor the largest of their operations, but if you are in the mood to shop around for gadgets old and new (it does feel just a little bit like new lamps for old) then you will find a happy hunting ground here. They have a coffee machine and you are welcome to browse.

So why this great enthusiasm of mine for Thorne? Well; although it is nearly 60 miles from the sea, it makes a good headquarters for anyone wanting to use and cruise the Ouse, the Trent and the Humber; it is suitably central for the Sheffield & South Yorkshire, the Aire & Calder and, through them, to the Leeds & Liverpool and the Calder & Hebble, neither of which is very far away. It offers, in its own inimitable style, such a range of eating, drinking and shopping delights that even a breakdown, enforcing a stay there, would afford plenty of compensations; and when it comes to looking after your boat, you couldn't be in a better place – and if your boat just happens to be a wooden one, everyone will be just that mite more pleased.

Leaving Thorne, you will pass the long stretch of moored boats by Stani-lands yard and marina; and the next two items to catch the eye are the old rail bridge and the new motorway bridge. After these, the canal continues its undramatic course with the River Don to the north, past Dunston Hill swing bridge until the remains of the lock appear on the right, where there is an easily overlooked boat pond tucked away – host to some quite unexpected craft. On the opposite bank, on the outskirts of Stainforth (except that Stainforth itself is really no more than outskirts) is the New Inn, with a pretty patch of grass to tempt you to moor outside (provided you don't draw much more than 3′). Stainforth (and its little sister on the other side, Fishlake) represents virtually the last outpost of civilisation before the canal meets the New Junction just after Bramwith Lock. The canal takes a sharp bend when it passes under the road bridge in the village, and it is wise to take extra precautions: slow down, and use the whistle. After the few attractive house fronts on both sides of the canal beyond the bridge, everything settles down to its usual quiet, uneventful pattern; until you arrive at the settlements a few cables before Bramwith bridge. Here you will find a run of farm buildings (one of which is graced by the O.S. map as a Hall), geese-a-flocking, goats-a-galloping and dogs forever barking. Like most bridges on this canal, it is operated on an extremely infor-mal basis: for example, once, in the middle of winter, I was asked to deliver the daily paper to the keeper of the lock a mile ahead; and you can regularly count on finding plenty of souls who are ready and willing to open not only their bridges but also their hearts to any sympathetic navigator.

Then comes the lock and after it a very popular spot for weekend barbecues, on the north bank just before the New Junction. It can be very busy; but dur-ing the week, especially out of season, it can feel remote – although you can see the Tom Puddings going along from the Sheffield & South Yorkshire into the New Junction for the trip along the Aire & Calder.

When it is your turn to decide whether to turn left (for Doncaster) or right (for Sykehouse) make sure that you pass well beyond the point before turning or keep well away from the south bank as there are shoal patches to both left and right. It is also appropriate now to begin to look out for the commercial traffic that uses these waterways. If there is anything special to watch out for, you will most probably be told by the keeper at Bramwith before you move on and out of the Stainforth & Keadby Canal.

BRAMWITH SWING BRIDGE	**BRAMWITH LOCK**
Bramwith,	Bramwith,
Doncaster,	Doncaster,
South Yorkshire	South Yorkshire
Restricting dimensions 22′ bank to bank	*Restricting dimensions* 215′ x 17′8″
Hand operated ●	*Rise and fall* 5′
Keeper operated ●	*Hand operated* ●
Facilities nearby None	*Keeper operated* ●
	Facilities nearby None
Remarks	*Remarks*
See Vazon Swing Bridge for opening times.	Vazon Swng Bridge for opening times.

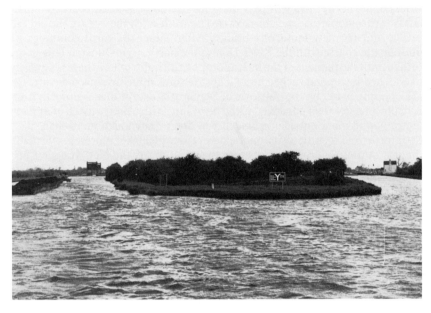

The Stainforth & Keadby on the right and the New Junction on the left – with a Tom Pudding on the way to Goole.

The New Junction

No-one would claim (not even BWB's most fervent supporters) that the New Junction Canal is a grand affair. It is neither so massive that it takes the breath away, nor so small that one marvels at it ever happening at all. Mercutio might perhaps anachronistically have been describing it: 'No, 'tis not so deep as a well, nor so wide as a churchdoor; but 'tis enough, 'twill serve.' In fact, it starts at Ordnance Survey grid reference 613 108 and runs in a generally northerly direction for just over 5 miles until it finds itself looking at the Southfield Reservoir on the other side of the Aire and Calder Navigation at grid reference 651 187.

So, the New Junction has no claim to being very long; and while it is deeper than the rest of the Sheffield & South Yorkshire system by a good 3' (bringing it up, or taking it down according to your point of view, to more than 13') that can hardly be calculated to win a prize for depth; and when it comes to width, it is true that two fairly beamy barges can pass in what might be called comfort, but it is also true that any craft finding itself between the two or between one of them and the bank would have little room for manoeuvre and not

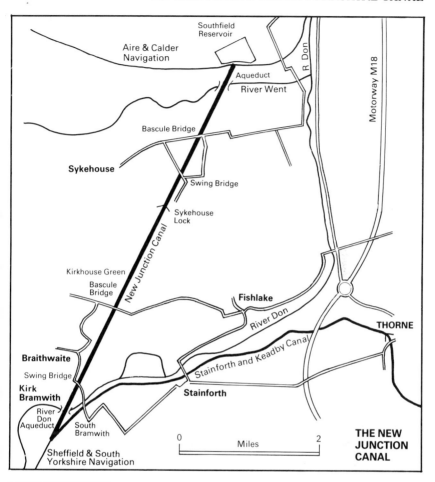

LOW LANE BRIDGE

Kirk Bramwith,
Doncaster,
South Yorkshire

Restricting dimensions 22' bank to bank.
Mechanised •
Keeper operated •
Facilities nearby None

Remarks
Opening times:
Monday to Thursday 0700-1730
Friday 0700-1630
Saturday 0700-1200
        1300-1700
Sunday 0900-1200
        1300-1700

TOP LANE BRIDGE

Top Lane,
Braithwaite,
Doncaster,
South Yorkshire

Restricting dimensions 22' bank to bank.
Mechanised •
Keeper operated •
Facilities nearby None

Remarks
See Low Lane Bridge for opening times.

KIRKHOUSE GREEN BRIDGE

Kirkhouse Green,
Doncaster,
South Yorkshire

Restricting dimensions   22' bank to bank.
Mechanised •
Keeper operated •
Facilities nearby
⌂
Hacienda. ½ mile. Closed all day Monday.

Remarks
See Low Lane Bridge for opening times.

SYKEHOUSE LOCK

Sykehouse Lock,
Goole,
North Humberside
☎ Thorne (0405) 85255
VHF channels 16 and 73

Restricting dimensions   300' x 22'
Rise and fall   7'
Mechanised •
Keeper operated •
Facilities nearby None

Remarks
See Low Lane Bridge for opening times.

KIRK LANE BRIDGE

Sykehouse,
Goole,
North Humberside

Restricting dimensions   22' bank to bank.
Mechanised •
Keeper operated •
Facilities nearby
⌂
Old George, Three Horseshoes. ½ mile.
S ½ mile (near pubs) General store.
☏ ½ mile
⚓

Remarks
See Low Lane Bridge for opening times.

SYKE HOUSE ROAD BRIDGE
As for Kirk Lane Bridge.

even a lot for survival. Nor, bearing in mind that some of our canals were cut by the Romans in the first century AD (for example, the Fossdyke from Torksey to Lincoln), can it by any stretch of the imagination be called old, since it was not opened until 1905. The purpose was to open up a connection between the Sheffield & South Yorkshire and the Aire & Calder, allowing Tom Puddings to get through with coal from Doncaster to Goole. However, it is as good as it needs to be and a darn sight better than it might be and it serves its traffic well. In fact, those who work the bridge (four in all) and the one lock are among the friendliest and most efficient I have come across over many years of encounters with hundreds of holders of similar office (some of whom are undoubtedly aware that Hamlet might actually have said: 'For who would bear the whips and scorns of time-keepers, the lock's delay, The insolence of office and the spurns That patient merit of the unworthy takes, When he himself might his own penning make with a bare windlass?'). They always seem to be ready and waiting, with the bridge fully open, just about 45 seconds before you actually reach the breach; not even in the foulest of weathers, have I been denied a friendly wave when passing through.

However, it is with no great feeling of warmth that I remember the very first time I ever poked *Valcon's* stem into the New Junction Canal: I was making my way from Keadby to Leeds on an extremely windy day in late autumn when the

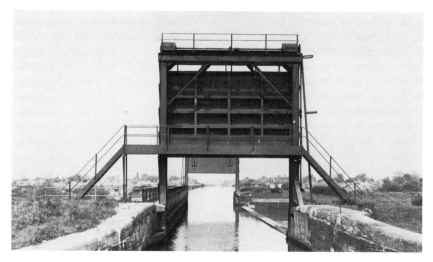

The Don Aqueduct on the New Junction Canal. Note the absence of any guard rail on the right of the waterway.

Beaufort scale was at a steady 8 and gusting at 10. I was due to turn into the canal after Bramwith Lock but had been asked to look out for a Tom Pudding on the move from Doncaster. The high winds were creating problems for the skipper, and the lock-keepers had been phoning ahead to try to keep his channel as clear as possible. While duly holding back once I had sighted him, I managed to drift onto a silt bank. I ungrounded myself without difficulty and the Tom Pudding went on its way with a generous acknowledgement from the skipper. I was at last free to point *Valcon's* bows in the general direction of the lock at Sykehouse; free, that is, except for the intervening edifice: the River Don aqueduct and the awesome aspect of its guillotine.

Although the whole amazing construction, built to prevent surging and flooding between the river and the canal in severely wet weather, was demonstrably strong enough to carry military tanks, let alone support a flood gate made entirely of steel, nevertheless I viewed it with the suspicion and approached it with the delicacy that I would accord to any Damoclean menace, symbolic or real. On its west side there is substantial girder work reaching well above water level; but on the east side the water laps on girders above which there is nothing, absolutely nothing at all. I found it disconcerting to note that the only things between me and the drop to the Don below were this single girder and the dozens of seagulls that were perched on it with all the insouciant confidence that only their ability to fly (and perhaps their total ignorance of Icarus) could remotely begin to justify. I told myself a good few times that traffic constantly used the aqueduct every day with none of the terrifying scenes of death and disaster that were flooding my mind, and so managed to coax myself back to the wheel and navigate the wretched thing.

Once past the monster, I relaxed, and the character of the canal appeared to change dramatically. While it would be misleading to suggest that I seemed to be surveying a land flowing with milk and honey, it would be extremely remiss not to refer to the general picturesqueness of the locality in enthusiastic terms: I find it one of the most attractive in the area. There are good vistas to be beheld from deck level (an unusual occurrence in the waterways of Lincolnshire and Yorkshire, this) and, in spite of the traffic on the canal and the all too obvious explosions of the wild-fowlers, there is still plenty of wild life with life, so with patience and a good pair of glasses there is more than enough to look at all along the five mile stretch.

Towards the north, Sykehouse Lock is a pleasure to negotiate, and the aqueduct that comes shortly after it is much less horrendous to contemplate than the one over the Don; on the other hand, it is not in such a good state of repair, and, since it spans the River Went, it is just too tempting to comment that it is not only 'went' but also 'gone.' At the end of the New Junction, just across the wide expanse of the Aire & Calder there is an even wider expanse (112 acres all told) that forms the Southfield reservoir. This reservoir has nothing at all to do with any domestic water supply; it was built in 1889 (and then enlarged between 1909 and 1914) as a pound for the canals, allowing the many pennings of craft along the navigation without unduly disturbing the levels or creating vast, disruptive surges at the opening and closing of the gates. Different from most back-up waters of this kind, its level is the same as that of the canal it serves, and not higher – held back by gates and impounding walls. It also makes it easier for the canal administrators and those at Goole docks to organise their supplies so that the level at Goole is maintained throughout; for there are not several docks with different levels at Goole, there is just one level, since all the docks are permanently interconnected. This reservoir is the headquarters of the Beaver Sailing Club (and they are extremely jealous guardians of what they call 'their sailing water') but there is no access from the canal side. (It may look as if it is possible to cruise across into it, but there is no way in, and the apparent entrances carry no water and are also foul at the bottom.)

Provided that you are not looking for sophisticated marinas, shops, French restaurants and the like, there is little doubt in my mind that in its five miles, the New Junction packs in more appeal that many other waterways that are, on a superficial assessment, bigger and better in every way. It is just unfortunate that BWB have not yet seen fit to create more good lay-bys (or just sound mooring spots, if only for the weekends) so that cruising folk can enjoy its delights even more than they can right now.

The Sheffield & South Yorkshire

After leaving the Stainforth & Keadby Canal and the last small lock for some considerable distance, you make a broad turn to the left, leaving the New Junction behind on the right, and make for the beginnings of some pretty unpretty industrial and commercial architecture. In fact, there are in the area some excellent examples of Victorian and *fin de siècle* industrial building design (for example, the canal basin at Sheffield, and also parts of Leeds, are inspired and inspiring works and only need somebody (or some body) to restore them to decency for them to be seen as the fantastic monuments that they are) but sadly, the approach to Doncaster displays some of the worst excesses of the Industrial Revolution let go into decay and some of the worst examples of modern industrial architecture that will stand very little chance of ever decaying since, like Tower Hamlets, they seem more likely to be destroyed by the spirit of their begetters.

LONG SANDALL LOCK

Long Sandall
Doncaster,
South Yorkshire

Restricting dimensions   243' x 22'
Rise and fall   11'
Mechanised   •
Keeper operated   •
Facilities nearby
⚓
100 yards upstream of lock.

Remarks
See Low Lane Bridge for opening times.

BARNBY DUN LIFT BRIDGE

Barnby Dun
Doncaster,
South Yorkshire
VHF channels 16 and 73

Restricting dimensions   22' bank to bank.
Mechanised   •
Keeper operated   •
Facilities nearby
⚓ 🚾
🍺 Star, 150 yards
S General and off-licence nearby
✉ 1 mile
✆ ½ mile

Remarks
See Low Lane Bridge for opening times.
Very busy road traffic at this bridge.

But take heart, all is not lost or overshadowed completely by poorly designed power stations. There are two oases before the centre of Doncaster: the small settlement of Barnby Dun (preceded by one of the new-style bascule bridges, as on the New Junction) where there are more than decent domestic and social facilities; and the lock at Long Sandall. In the days of keeper Hubert Allen, this lock was pre-eminent in the annals of canals for its well-kept surrounds and gardens; but now the prize crown for best-kept locks goes elsewhere and the competition to gain one of the coveted moorings just by the lock itself is no longer as fierce as it used to be. These two spots are worth noting and savouring for there is little else to charm until well after the lock in Doncaster.

In mediaeval times, there was an extensive system of natural river navigations that served the inland trade of Yorkshire. Perhaps the busiest of those in 'olden times' was the River Idle (pp. 97-101) which was navigable from the town (and then, of course, port!) of Bawtry into the River Trent at Stockwith. Another natural navigation, although much more difficult and hazardous, was the River Don but only downstream of Doncaster. In the early days, the trade on the River Don was quite small and in no way helped by the construction in the early 17th century of the 'Dutch' River drainage channel. One of the old

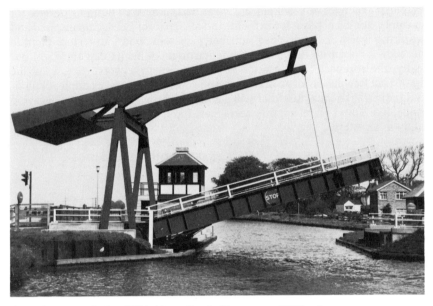

A very busy spot: the 'new' lift bridge at Barnby Dun, now on VHF radio.

outfalls of the River Don, into the River Aire near Snaith and Cowick, where some of the old river can still be inspected, was navigable until the end of the 17th century, when the previously moveable bridge near the outfall was permanently fixed during repairs.

The first attempts to make the River Don navigable as far as the industrialised area around Rotherham and Sheffield were made in 1697, but were unsuccessful. In 1731, boats managed to reach Aldwarke; and by 1740 got as far as Rotherham. In 1751, the navigation was open to Tinsley, from which point on there was a toll road to Sheffield. The lowest part of the River Don Navigation (which used the Dutch River, always a dangerous navigation then and now) was improved by the addition of the Stainforth and Keadby canal, providing access to the River Trent at Keadby. Immediately after the wars with Napoleon, the canal was extended from Tinsley into the heart of Sheffield and in 1905, as we have seen earlier, the New Junction was opened to make the connection with the much more financially successful Aire & Calder.

However, improvement did not end there, and, nearly 80 years later, another betterment scheme was completed: the length of the South Yorkshire Canal between Rotherham and Bramwith, a distance of 22 miles, and also the New Junction. Over this length, a short stretch in Rotherham consists of natural river, but from Rotherham Lock to Eastwood Lock, the navigation is an artificial channel. From there, the navigation follows the natural river course to Kilnhurst Flood Lock where it again enters an artificial channel, continuing through Swinton and the two locks at Mexborough to follow the natural river course again for a distance of 7 miles to Doncaster. It then rejoins an artificial channel through Long Sandall Lock for another 7 miles where it then meets with the head of the New Junction.

The scheme involved the lengthening, improvement or reconstruction of 10 locks, the widening or removal of 8 bridges, the major realignment of navigation channels at 4 sites and the reduction of sharp curves and any other restrictions to larger craft between Doncaster and Rotherham. Thus, at a cost of £16 million, barges of up to 700 tonnes are now able to reach Rotherham. However, in spite of the modernisation, when I took *Valcon* up the section to see the changes for myself, I was held up for ages in the teeth of a gale of rain and hail while the electrics and mechanics were being fettled up by a peripatetic engineer. Later experience of the rest of the betterment showed that this hold-up was a false omen, for the rest have worked faultlessly whenever I have needed to pass along the system.

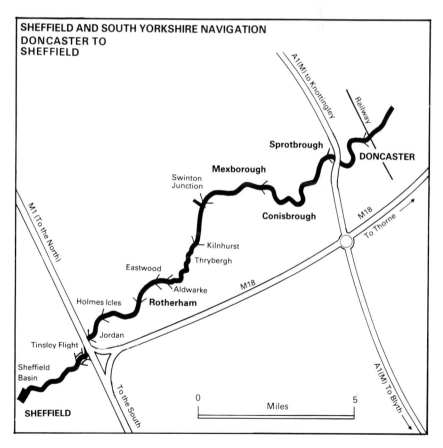

Doncaster looms ahead for apparent ages; and not even the boat owners of Strawberry Island have been able to ameliorate the unpleasantness of this approach. The club here is a thriving one, and members are to be encountered all over the system covered by this volume. I have never been able to find a channel for *Valcon* (needing six feet plus) that didn't suggest I might be looking for trouble when the intention was to look for a haven; so I have not myself been able to taste the delights of the intriguingly named island. And havens are not easy to come across in this soft under-belly run through what was at one time a generous, prosperous, good-looking town. Actually, its 'soft under-belly' is really more akin to the roofworks of an armadillo, since the collection of ugly hardware that goes to make up much of the girderwork of the bridges is a positive indictment to those who perpetrated it and those who permitted them so to do.

If you can make arrangements and if your draught permits, do stay at Strawberry Island rather than risk any other, closer and apparently more convenient mooring. There are places near the lock itself (where the keeper now works from a glass-enclosed office which seems wholly taken up by a vast desk that is completely surrounded by audio/visual aids that indicate the state of the lock and its attendant waters) and I was once foolhardy enough to stay overnight at a tempting-looking site just by the railway bridge. The bridge itself is a real hazard to anyone walking underneath it on the sides of the canal, for there are low-hanging protrusions that are extremely difficult to see and that will bring you up with a vengeance if you should overlook or forget them. The bridge was not the only cause for alarm (literally!) for I am sure that no traveller on the Inter City 125s that rush north and south are aware of the stunning confusion they are creating below. (*Kings II ix 20:* 'The driving is like the driving of Jehu the son of Nimshi; for he driveth furiously.') Finally, heaping Pelion upon Ossa in a most savage way, *Valcon* was cast off with her ropes cut, my gear dumped in the canal and the Avon dinghy slashed. I had had a similar experience in the middle of the night in the middle of Rotherham; and if that doesn't bring to mind an image to conjure with, then nothing on this section will upset you. It was about 0300 (not my best time at all) that I heard banging and shouting. Anthea and I were living on board at the time, and therefore ready to investigate any sound that boded ill for us or for *Valcon*. By the time we were on deck, it was too late to do anything but observe how our ropes had been slashed and all our accessible gear dumped in the canal. When we got ourselves organised we found we had drifted a good two cables towards the lock gates – but just managing not to have caught on any of the many overhanging coal hoists and similar devices and traps for the unwary. However, I can hear the learned now say, 'That was Rotherham: you ought to have known what to expect', and it is true that Rotherham possesses neither a reputation nor an environment that can be called salubrious; but surely the same cannot be said in such strict terms about Doncaster?

Moving through the lock itself is indeed a pleasure even for those boaters who never knew it in its primeval prime. Shortly after, on the north bank the

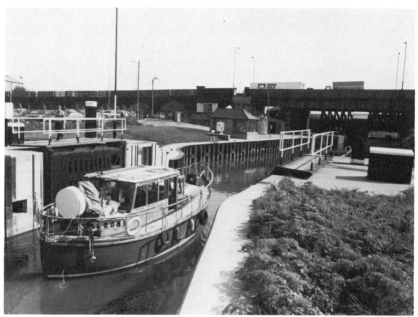

Doncaster is hardly recognisable after the modernisation, improvement and refurbishing scheme along this waterway. Mooring just outside the lock, both above and below, is possible – but guards should be set!

DONCASTER LOCK

Marshgate,
Doncaster,
South Yorkshire

Remarks
See Low Lane Lock for opening times

Restricting dimensions   315' x 22'
Rise and fall   5'
Mechanised   •
Keeper operated   •
Facilities nearby

✕ 🖵 ½ mile to town. Many pubs and restaurants.
  S ½ mile to town. Excellent facilities.
✉ ½ mile to town.
  ♪ Nearest in town.   ⚓ below lock

river reunites with the canal and there is also a bay that is usually busy with commercial traffic. The next item of interest comes with the great bend at Hexthorpe. This has now been improved and swings broadly round to port, leaving ahead an area that can look as if it is part of the navigable waterway; but take care if there is a touch of fog, and watch the signs: Keep Left. It is after this bend that the waterway takes upon itself a completely unexpected character, becoming one of the prettiest stretches that I know. The first sign is the landing stage for the Doncaster water bus that operates during the season.

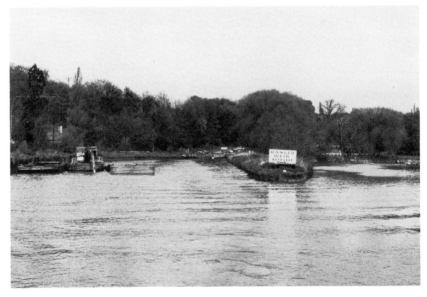

The approach to Sprotbrough Lock from upstream. The weir is fiercish.

From there on the scenery becomes steeply wooded and lush in a way that invites the word idyllic. In addition, there are some equally unexpected views of dramatic building: just before Sprotbrough you will get some stunning sights of the apparently impossible feats of architecture that went into the creation of the bridges and the viaduct. Of all the places in the northeast waterways region for a camera, this must be a prime contender whether you prefer colour transparencies or plain, old-fashioned steam black and white. Sadly there are no places where you easily get to the side or attach your craft to the banks; but this becomes of little importance when you note that you are no distance at all from one of the most favoured, but still not over-popularised, over-populated or exploited, spots on the system: Sprotbrough. It is at this lock that the keeper, Dennis Petty, has won the Castleford Area prize in the national lock competition; as well as the special memorial Hubert Allen (once of Long Sandall fame) trophy.

The *genius loci* of Sprotbrough must have a hard time of it deciding precisely where to hang up its hat, strike root or drop anchor since the charms of the place are almost equally divided between the urban, the arboreal and the riparian.

In the face of such a polarity of choices, I decided to ignore the extremes and settle for the mainstream in the form of Main Street. Here, not quite clustered around a crossroads that doesn't and not quite embraced by a square that isn't is to be found Sprotbrough's closest approximation to a nucleus.

SPROTBROUGH LOCK

Sprotbrough,
Doncaster,
South Yorkshire

Restricting dimensions   234' x 21'
Rise and fall   6'
Mechanised   ●
Keeper operated   ●
Facilities nearby
⚓ ⚓
🏠 Ivanhoe Hotel. 1 mile.
S   1 mile
✉ 1 mile

Remarks
See Low Lane Lock for opening times.
Landing stage below lock

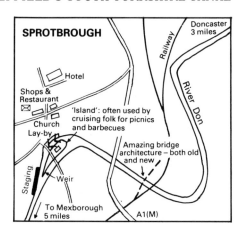

Here is the church with the rare and strangely carved stone chair in its dim and shadowy chancel – not accessible to the chance visitor. Here is the post office, doing its best to look like any ordinary cottage with no claim to fame except for the apparent last minute thought of its legend. Here is the village 'hall', where it seemed possible to get afternoon tea at any time of day, albeit in the absence of any apparent clientele of any kind. And here also is the village arcade, that is not quite Arcadian and certainly not arcane.

For those who like to socialise, but in small groups and in a rural setting; for those with a non-topiarian love of trees and an addiction to thickly wooded slopes; and for those whose taste is for a riverside by waters that are harnessed and controlled, there can surely be no location better equipped to indulge their pleasures.

Not only is Sprotbrough without an obvious centre or singular essence, it is also something of an enigma and an oasis. In terms of nomenclature it comes off pretty poorly when compared with two of its close neighbours: Warmsworth and Loversall. 'Warm' and 'Love' have both got to be that much more appealing than 'Sprot'. On the other hand, it must also be compared in a different way with its other neighbours; those monumental symbols to man's industrial insanity such as Mexborough, Conisbrough and Rotherham and that lets Doncaster, for which at least part of Sprotbrough is a dormitory, off lightly. For miles the general surroundings are degenerate and there is a drab and dreary appearance to the vast majority of buildings, all of which have suffered directly from accession and accretion of coal mines and slag heaps. Only the local magnesium of Conisbrough Castle has been sublime enough to stay clean and pure in the dirty, dust-defiled atmosphere.

Fortunately, none of this outrage seriously mars the pretty village of Sprotbrough and its environs; although many of its trees bear leaves that are a whiter shade of green as a result of the pale powders of pollution that can still cloud the atmosphere. Sprotbrough is supposed to have been so appealing and inspiring that Sir Walter Scott was moved to conceive and write part of *Ivanhoe*

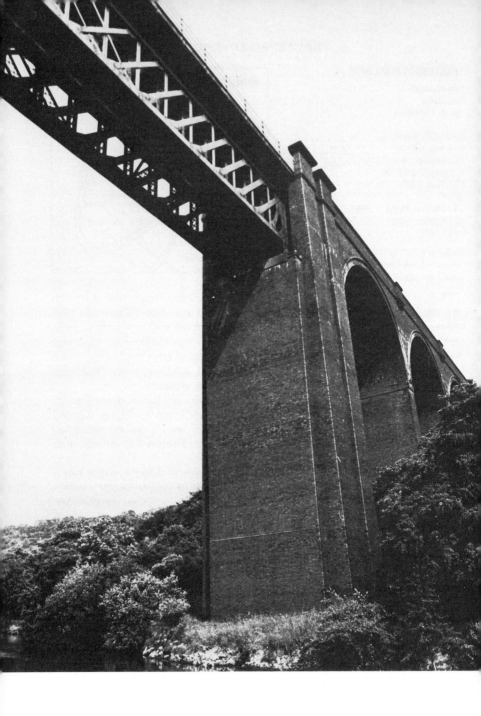

Between Doncaster and Conisbrough the bridges and viaducts are impressive.

here. Indeed, once you turn your back on the village itself and wander down to the refurbished lock and the mooring jetties at the bottom of the hill, it is easy to forget everything but the ferocious looking weir and the still-black or spume-white waters that there combine to invest the tree-bedecked valley with a veritable aura of magic and mystery.

None of these delights to the senses and the imagination is really spoiled by the fact that there is a car park here, as well as the staging point for the water bus. It is actually a spot well chosen for any sort of transport of delight. And when the need for a potion more potent than water overcomes the call of the Don, it is not a long walk up the hill and through the village to the Ivanhoe Hotel, where their mental refreshments are as good as their food and drink. Here was I told the tale of the cricketing Richard Lumb for whom the Ivanhoe was home until the family sold out; and here was I reliably informed that Douglas Bader's father . . . grandfather . . . and uncle were, at one and the same time and person, the vicar of the church. Other reliable sources told me that Douglas Bader had once spent a holiday there . . . they thought!

However, there was nothing but first-hand information from the landlord himself: 'I'll tell you before you ask me. Yes, I am one of the Irish Burkes. He was executed in Edinburgh 1829. We're even in the dictionary.' And so he was: 'to burke' is a transitive verb meaning to murder in such a way as to leave no mark on the body; usually by suffocation.

Sprotbrough is not likely to mark your person either; it may well take your breath away, but it will certainly not harm you. Much more is it likely to charm you.

And then, in no time at all, it is time for all change; for it is not far upriver from Sprotbrough that you will enter a kind of valley of despair (or slough of despond) that will lead you to Mexborough. Expectation at this time must surely be running low for any boater who has not been this way before; but the betterment men have been here and an excellent job they have done. The lock has always lifted boats into a plateau of a canal, and it has no doubt always afforded good views in so far as height usually does. But now there is a difference: where before there were pit heaps and stacks and huge cooling towers, there is now an agreeably landscaped vista; and where before the lock had been ugly to look at and difficult to enter, Mexborough Top Lock now offers ease of access, a decent mooring spot and plenty of facilities. In particular, there is a welcoming pub close by, and a string of shops along the nearby main road; and it is not far to the supermarkets of Mexborough's town centre, an experience not to omit.

There is only one minor hazard anywhere near either Mexborough Low or Mexborough Top Lock, and that is just outside the Low Lock where, if you are at all underpowered, the river can, at times, take you unawares by its unexpected power. After the Top Lock, there comes quite an eerie view of the Don running along many feet beneath the canal to the south. Then comes the major improvement at Double Bridges which has worked extremely well. It used to be a case of all hands to the wheel and all eyes to the front for it was quite a demanding operation manoeuvring through the blind bends, but now it is all sweetness and light.

Then on to Swinton Lock, as everyone still insists on calling it, where there are signs of busy activity everywhere, thanks mainly to the traffic of the family firm of Ernest Waddington Ltd. It can be difficult for pleasure craft to find a way through the apparent maze of huge barges that are arrayed and rafted in what looks like a solid battle formation. The biggest by far is Waddingtons' *Confidence*, made from the fore part of one barge joined to the aft section of another, complete with a new strengthened middle section. This unusual carrier was made specially to transport four 333-tonne castings from Goole to Doncaster, one at a time, and to undertake similar return journeys.

There is no doubt that the heart of Swinton is in the bosom of the Waddington family. Indeed, so impressed have been British Waterways by their efforts over the years, that in April 1982, Sir Frank Price, the then chairman, conducted a ceremony at the Swinton Lock to rename it Waddington Lock, to recognise the 'long and enthusiastic association with the Navigation and neighbouring waterways' that has been the life of Victor Waddington. It was not long after this event that the two locks at Eastwood became one flesh through the betterment and reconstruction programme and were renamed: this time after Sir Frank himself. His retirement was indeed well marked by the naming of names.

Then on to Kilnhurst where the river joins again and then to Aldwarke where it leaves. Care is needed when working these locks as the configuration of the banks and the conjoining of the waters does not make itself completely clear at first glance. However, it is not difficult to remember that the river joins the navigation from the left just outside Kilnhurst, where there is an impressive weir, and leaves it to the left just before Aldwarke. Here, there is a good mooring station and a pretty stone bridge.

There are one or two fair visions before Rotherham, and it must be said that the new locks do make progress both smooth and problem free, so there really is plenty of time to float, if not actually stand as Davies would have us do, and stare. But it is not long before it begins to come clear that it is not going to come clean again. Right up to Rotherham, one might claim that 'fings ain't wot they used to be', but once arrived, it is made abundantly manifest that 'fings' are exactly what they used to be or perhaps just a little bit worse.

Once past the stretches improved for commercial use, the whole canal picture begins to disintegrate, and the waterway itself and its adjacent canal corridor are depressingly inefficient. The first lock inside Rotherham is indicative of what is to come: the mechanics are not in good order; there is seldom the depth of water there is supposed to be; and it is generally not possible to moor alongside the banks because of the lack of water and the presence of unwanted presents in the form of beds, mattresses, tyres, fan belts, prams, and all kinds of wire: chicken, barbed, fencing, telephone and almost any kind you may care to mention except live wire, for in very truth every single thing in the canal seems dead. All this is indeed a pity, since there are comprehensive facilities to

MEXBOROUGH LOW LOCK

c/o Post Office,
Denaby Main,
South Yorkshire

Restricting dimensions 234' x 21'
Rise and fall 10'
Mechanised •
Keeper operated •
Facilities nearby None.

Remarks
Opening times:
Monday-Thursday 0800-1200 hours
1230-1630 hours
Friday 0800-1200 hours
1230-1530 hours
Saturday 0700-1200 hours
1300-1700 hours
Sunday 0900-1200 hours
1300-1700 hours
Landing stage below lock.

WADDINGTON LOCK

Dun Street,
Swinton,
Mexborough,
South Yorkshire

Restricting dimensions 234' x 21'
Rise and fall 6'
Mechanised •
Keeper operated •
Facilities nearby
🎣
🍽 Red House Hotel. 400 yards.
S 400 yards.
✉ 1 mile.
♪ ½ mile.

Remarks
Short-stay moorings, 1 mile upstream of this
lock, at Wharfe Road, Kilnhurst. New facility.
See Mexborough Low Lock for opening times.

MEXBOROUGH TOP LOCK

New Top Lock House,
Church Street,
Mexborough,
South Yorkshire

Restricting dimensions 234' x 21'
Rise and fall 6'
Mechanised •
Keeper operated •
Facilities nearby
🎣
🍽 Ferry Boat Inn. 200 yards
S 600 yards
✉ 600 yards

Remarks
See Mexborough Low Lock for opening times.
Landing stage below lock.

KILNHURST LOCK

Kilnhurst,
South Yorkshire

Restricting dimensions 234' x 21'
Rise and fall 9"
Mechanised •
Keeper operated •
Facilities nearby None.
🎣
Remarks
Short-stay moorings, ½ mile downstream of
this lock, at Wharfe Road, Kilnhurst. New
facility.
See Mexborough Low Lock for opening times.

hand in the city centre including an excellent Chinese restaurant and the prison-cum-chapel on the bridge. The first is straightforward and delivers what you expect from a decent cuisine, but the second is anything but straightforward, being surrounded by myth and legend with a combination of characters and tales that defy the imagination. If you can ignore the canal and its delinquency, there is a lot to be said for exploring from here.

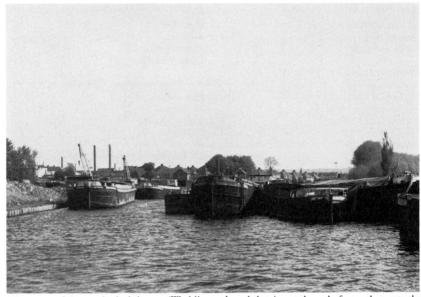

The name of the nearby lock is now 'Waddington'; and that is not the only factor that puts the stamp of this company on the locality. Proceed with caution; happily there are men and barges at work!

ALDWARKE LOCK

Aldwarke,
Rotherham,
South Yorkshire

Restricting dimensions   234' x 21'
Rise and fall   5'6"
Mechanised   •
Keeper operated   •
Facilities nearby
⚓
Remarks
See Mexborough Low Lock for opening times.

FRANK PRICE LOCK

Eastwood,
Rotherham,
South Yorkshire

Restricting dimensions   234' x 21'
Rise and fall 11'6"
Mechanised   •
Keeper operated   •
Facilities nearby
⚓
Remarks
See Mexborough Low Lock for opening times.

ROTHERHAM LOCK

Rotherham,
South Yorkshire

Restricting dimensions   62' x 16'
Rise and fall   2'
Hand operated   •
Boater operated   •
Windlass required   •
Facilities nearby
🛒 ✉ S ✆
Remarks
Rotherham town, 2 minutes walk for all facilities.

ICKLES LOCK

Rotherham,
South Yorkshire

Restricting dimensions   62' x 16'
Rise and fall   6'6"
Hand operated   •
Boater operated   •
Windlass required   •
Facilities nearby
None.

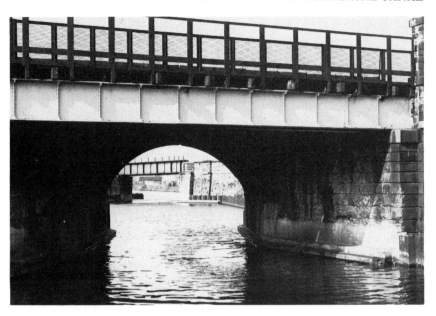

Double Bridges – after its conversion . . . and the new bridgeworks by the neighbouring power station chimneys.

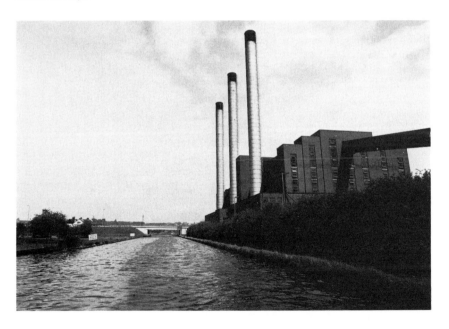

HOLMES LOCK

Holmes Lock,
Off Salter Lane,
Holmes Lane,
Rotherham,
South Yorkshire

Restricting dimensions 62' x 16'
Rise and fall 9'10"
Hand operated •
Boater operated •
Windlass required •
Facilities nearby
None.
Remarks
No lock-keeper in attendance.

JORDAN LOCK

Rotherham,
Yorkshire

Restricting dimensions 62' x 16'
Rise and fall 1'6"
Hand operated •
Boater operated •
Windlass required •
Facilities nearby
None.
Remarks
No lock-keeper in attendance.

Ahead lie plenty of dismal sights and scenes as ugliness takes over completely. But there are two compensatory experiences to be enjoyed in the splendid achievements of the Tinsley Flight of locks into Sheffield, and the Canal Basin at the head of navigation in Sheffield. However, there is still a lot of grot in between and some quite hard work if you are to achieve the sanctuary of the basin. From the top of the Tinsley Flight of locks to the Canal Basin is 3 miles of industrial horror; the canal forming a ribbon of unexpectedly orange, green and yellow water that cuts a wary course through thick weed and a variety of floating and submerged inland flotsam and jetsam: from huge polythene bags and cast-off clothing, to fan belts and bicycle frames, to stolen television sets and abandoned motor cars. The slim waterway is the only pleasant feature in the otherwise darkly satanic back alleyway of the Industrial Revolution's mercantile mills. (The mills of God may grind slowly and exceeding small; but the mills of Man grow swiftly, and they grow exceeding tall.)

The Tinsley Flight now consists of 11 locks. It used to be 12 but the old numbers 7 and 8 were combined in 1959 into a new concrete chamber, with a rise of 12', to enable the construction of a low railway bridge that would still permit decent air draught, or 'briggage' as it is known hereabouts, to boat traffic. The flight drops, in the words of keeper Jim Bradley, 'a heavy 96' in a short one and a half miles' from the top of the lock to the river. The locks to watch out for especially are No. 6 and No. 11 counting from the top. If you draw more than 3', it is advisable to put in at least another foot of water from the previous lock. There is a severe shortage of water in the last pound and the miniature channel through it (it looks like a small lake!) is tortuous. In addition, the sills of 6 and 11 can cause problems to anyone who is not patient enough to wait for water or to make an exit at dead slow ahead.

When coming up at night, it is essential to make sure that both lock gates are closed behind you and that all paddles, cloughs or sluices are shut as tightly as possible. There are three reasons for this: all the water for the flight has to be pumped up from the river to No. 1 lock; the whole flight has been stocked with fish by the British Waterways Board and a number of local angling clubs; and

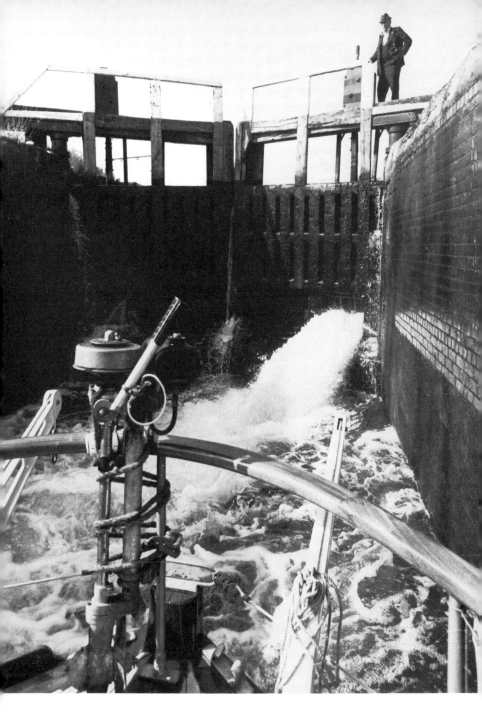

The bottom of the Tinsley Flight .

Plumpers Lock (No. 9) is used by the Tinsley Wire Company for their commercial water supply.

The lock-keeper likes one or two days' notice of your arrival so that he can fill up all the pounds and also arrange to be available to help work the locks. (The best time I have ever managed in *Valcon* was a two hour stint going down; and that was with the help of a crew of two, the lock-keeper and the pump attendant. The way up is a long, hard, haul.) There is no doubt that the Tinsley Flight, in many places, is an impressive sight, even one approaching a certain kind of grandeur, and it is always an energetic experience. The last one and a half miles before the basin need to be taken very slowly, for there is little water except in the middle of the channel and any speed at all will pull away the sides, and the fabric is already in poor shape.

Once inside the canal basin however, there is much to create interest. What it actually looks like, contrasts so vividly with what might be, that one can stand mesmerised by ambivalence: anger at those who have let it all go by the board; and keen support and sympathy for those who want to refurbish so that it can stand proud and useful once more, gracing the city with an historic yet up-to-date aesthetic amenity. All being well, by the end of the decade British Waterways Board and the Sheffield city council will have made the approach canal an enjoyable trip (with a depth of at least two metres) and the basin itself the centre of leisure, pleasure, enterprise and craft. All the public bodies that are in any way concerned with the development say they are extremely keen for the canal and the basin to 'come good' again, but it really is time that deeds took over from say-so, for precisely the same things were being said and precisely the same excuses and blames were being made and laid when I wintered in the basin nearly ten years ago. However, at least a start has been made on the cottages and the arches. A major refurbishment attack by the City Council has got them, together with the periphery and general environment of the basin into better fettle, and more is planned when the city fathers and the Board's administrators get their heads together sympathetically . . . and the money becomes available.

TINSLEY FLIGHT (12 LOCKS)

Tinsley,
Sheffield,
South Yorkshire

Restricting dimensions 62' x 16'
Rise and fall 6'6" (No. 7; 11'6")
Hand operated •
Boater operated •
Windlass required •
Facilities nearby
None.

Remarks
No overnight moorings between locks.
Boatmen are requested to seek the assistance and advice of the lengthsman when negotiating the Tinsley Flight. ☎ Sheffield (0742) 441981.
Lock No. 10: Small shopping area ½ mile, all facilities.

END-PIECE

The canal and basin received their grand opening on Monday 22 February, 1819, in front of nearly 60,000 people. The local press, *The Iris*, in a rush of purple ink to paper, put it this way:' . . . the inhabitants of that town have vainly wished and attempted to break down the barriers of invidious separation which have held them imprisoned in the heart of their district like as many miners who by a fall of rubbish are secluded in a subterranean abyss, to which their companions have to force a passage within a yard or two of their retreat when a few strokes of the pickaxe would have set them free at liberty and restored them to the air and the light of heaven.' Let us hope that some ghostly reporter of that strangely named publication will be around for the next release and restoration.

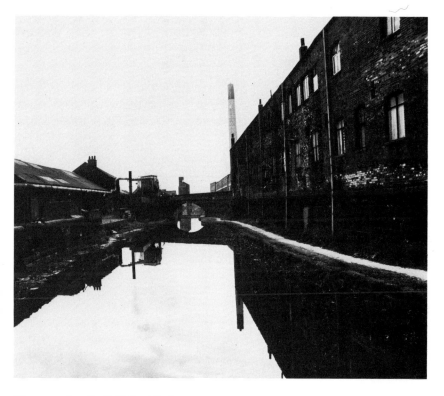

The approach to Sheffield Canal Basin.

IV. THE AIRE & CALDER NAVIGATION

The Aire & Calder Navigation is one of our premier commercial waterways, and has been the subject of consistent improvement since the first craft ever reached Leeds and Wakefield in 1700. The waterway is based upon the Rivers Aire and Calder, but over the centuries several completely artificial sections have been built to avoid difficult stretches of river. The navigation was nationalised along with most of Britain's inland waterways in 1948, and since 1962 improvements (lengthening of locks and deepening of the channel) have increased the maximum size of craft able to use the system from 320 to 500 tons, Goole to Leeds.

The main line runs from the Port of Goole on the River Ouse to Castleford and then splits, the main line continuing to Leeds, while the Wakefield section (River Calder) gives access to that town and to the Calder and Hebble Navigation. The Leeds & Liverpool Canal connects at Leeds. The Selby Canal connects at Knottingley, while the New Junction Canal connects with the Sheffield & South Yorkshire Navigation. From Goole to Leeds, the maximum craft dimensions must seem daunting to the skipper of a small GRP cruiser, for they are: 182' x 18' x 8' x 14' (air draught). None of the distances in the system is massive, nor are there very many locks. These are the details:

Goole-Castleford:	24 miles. 3 locks. 1 flood lock	
Castleford-Wakefield:	8 miles. 4 locks. 3 flood locks	
	(this includes ½ mile on the Calder & Hebble)	
Castleford-Leeds:	10 miles. 6 locks. 2 flood locks	
Selby-Knottingley:	11¾ miles. 3 locks. 1 flood lock	

Goole to Castleford

There is little to do with the Aire & Calder Navigation that is not connected with Goole; and there is little to do with Goole that is not directly associated with the Aire & Calder. Their connection with one another goes back a long time and is partly tied to another important Yorkshire waterway, the River Don.

The Dutch River empties into the River Ouse at Goole. It is, in fact, no more nor less than an immense open drain but it is also a continuation of the River Don from a point close to East Cowick. The River Don originally joined the River Aire near Rawcliffe, and even today its old course can still be seen and traced to Eskamhorn. The man-made channels were all part of the great drainage scheme of Cornelius Vermuyden, the famous Dutch engineer who in 1626 obtained a grant from the Crown for one third of all the land he recovered. The

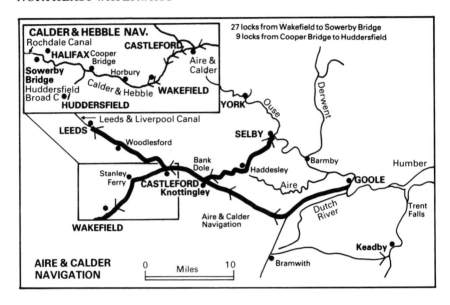

AIRE AND CALDER NAVIGATION

Distances
Leeds to Goole 34 miles
Wakefield to Goole 31 miles (Aire & Calder)
Bank Dole to Selby 12 miles (Selby Canal)
Wakefield to Sowerby Bridge 21 miles (Calder
   & Hebble Canal)
Non-tidal throughout.

Dimensions
Aire & Calder
   Length 130'
   Beam 17'
   Draught 7'
   Air draught 12'
Selby
   Length 70'
   Beam 16'
   Draught 4'
   Air draught 10'
Calder & Hebble
   Length 57'6" (120' to Broad Cut)
   Beam 14'2" (17'6" to Broad Cut)
   Draught 5' (6'6" to Broad Cut)
   Air draught 9' (11' to Broad Cut)

Locks
Aire & Calder 13 (+4 on the Wakefield arm)
Selby 4
Calder & Hebble 39

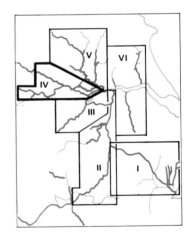

Traffic
The Aire & Calder is thick with substantial commercial traffic. The Calder & Hebble is used greatly by narrow boats and light pleasure craft; but the Selby is used little by only quite small craft.

Remarks
The Selby Canal is silting up through lack of use. It is essential to keep to a central course and it is difficult to turn for any craft over 30'.

OS Maps (1:50,000)
104 Leeds & Bradford
105 York
111 Sheffield & Doncaster
110 Sheffield and Huddersfield

Passage may be requested through manned locks and moveable bridges outside the opening hours (commonly referred to as 'call out') by telephoning the Freight Manager's (North) Office at Leeds (0532) 771804. Requests should be telephoned not later than 1500 hours for passage later on the day in question or not later than 12 noon on Friday for weekend requirements. Although every effort will be made to satisfy such requests, no guarantee can be given that requests can be accepted automatically.

Calder and Hebble Locks – Handspikes
Boatmen are reminded that they must have a handspike to operate the unusual type of clough (sluice) gear which exists at some of the locks on this canal. During times of high river flows a number of flood gates are closed and are impassable until levels recede. Boatmen should, therefore, check with Castleford Flood Lock (☎ Castleford (0977) 554351) or the Section Inspector at Mirfield (☎ Mirfield (0924) 492151) before entering the navigation.

Indicator boards, marked in green, yellow and red inform the boatman about prevailing conditions regarding flood levels. Their instructions must be obeyed at all times. Within the GREEN level: safe to proceed; within the YELLOW level: proceed with caution; with in the RED level: do not proceed.

Huddersfield Broad Canal
All locks are operated by boatmen who should be equipped with a Leeds and Liverpool Canal type windlass which can be used also to operate Turnbridge Locomotive liftbridge. Assistance can be sought from the canalman at Red Doles Lock (☎ Huddersfield (0484) 36732).

Navigation authority
British Waterways Board,
Castleford Area,
Lock Lane,
Castleford WF10 2LH
☎ (0977) 554351/5

Water authority
Yorkshire Water,
21 Park Square South,
Leeds LS1 2QG.
☎ (0532) 440191

area from Goole to Hatfield was overrun by Dutch and Flemish settlers and French exiles all engaged in reclaiming 24,000 acres of marshlands. The English farmers around Thorne and Fishlake complained that the drains being cut by the settlers flushed the river and caused it to overflow, thus ruining their crops. Wild scenes of riot and rebellion ensued, with the result that Vermuyden cut the Dutch River channel in order to relieve the River Don and draw off its waters more rapidly.

At about the same time, Selby was known as 'ye place on ye Ouze to wich most goods either imported from abroade or to be exported thither are now brought.' However, shortly after, the Rivers Aire and Calder were opened to navigation for small vessels and trade through Selby declined. In 1778, the canal from the Aire at Haddlesey to Selby was opened and trade picked up until the real challenge came with the opening of the Goole to Knottingley Canal, which omitted Selby altogether and made water access much easier from the river to Sheffield and South Yorkshire. The exit at Goole was below the more difficult reaches of the river and, while a site below Swinefleet would have cut out two more difficult bends, it could not be built so far down because of the Dutch River.

TABLE OF DISTANCES

	Goole	Rawcliffe Bridge	New Junction Canal	Heck Basin	Bank Dole Junction	Haddlesey	Selby	Castleford Junction	Woodlesford	Leeds	Stanley Ferry	Wakefield Fall Ing	Dewsbury	Cooper Bridge	Huddersfield	Halifax	Sowerby Bridge
Goole		4	8	12	17	23	28	24	29	34	29	31	39	44	47	50	52
Rawcliffe Bridge	4		4	8	13	19	24	20	25	30	25	27	35	40	43	46	48
New Junction Canal	8	4		4	9	15	20	16	21	26	21	23	31	36	39	42	44
Heck Basin	12	8	4		5	11	16	12	17	22	17	19	27	32	35	38	40
Bank Dole Junction	17	13	9	5		6	11	7	12	17	12	14	22	27	30	33	35
Haddlesey	23	19	15	11	6		5	13	18	23	18	20	28	33	36	39	41
Selby	28	24	20	16	11	5		18	23	28	28	30	33	38	41	44	46
Castleford Junction	24	20	16	12	7	13	18		5	10	5	7	15	20	23	26	28
Woodlesford	29	25	21	17	12	18	23	5		5	10	12	20	25	28	31	33
Leeds	34	30	26	22	17	23	28	10	5		15	17	25	30	33	36	38
Stanley Ferry	29	25	21	17	12	18	28	5	10	15		2	10	15	18	21	23
Wakefield Fall Ing	31	27	23	19	14	20	30	7	12	17	2		8	13	16	19	21
Dewsbury	39	35	31	27	22	28	33	15	20	25	10	8		5	8	11	13
Cooper Bridge	44	40	36	32	27	33	38	20	25	30	15	13	5		3	6	8
Huddersfield	47	43	39	35	30	36	41	23	28	33	18	16	8	3		3	5
Halifax	50	46	42	38	33	39	44	26	31	36	21	19	11	6	3		2
Sowerby Bridge	52	48	44	40	35	41	46	28	33	38	23	21	13	8	5	2	

Until July 1862, when the Aire & Calder Company completed the canal to Goole and also opened the docks, Goole was a modest, if not indeed insignificant, village on the south side of the Dutch River; the part that is now referred to as Olde Goole. The church of St. John, built in 1849, was erected on a piece of land donated by the Aire & Calder Navigation Company, and they also carried much of the building materials free of charge. So, the town grew up around the canal, and has, more or less, been devoted to it ever since. Plans for the docks and town were put into the hands of George Leather and John Rennie; but Rennie died in 1821 and the completion of the whole scheme was left to Leather.

For those who approach Goole for the first time, with their previous experience of locks being (say) Naburn or some of the hand-operated types on the Stainforth & Keadby, or even the nearly automatics on the Sheffield & South Yorkshire, the locks in this inland part will come as something of a surprise if not indeed a shock and a threat. They are massive; and for any novice boating family in a small GRP cabin cruiser must (when they meet them for the first time, perhaps in the company of a barge, a tug and a coaster) make them think twice about going through with the penning procedure. In fact, they look

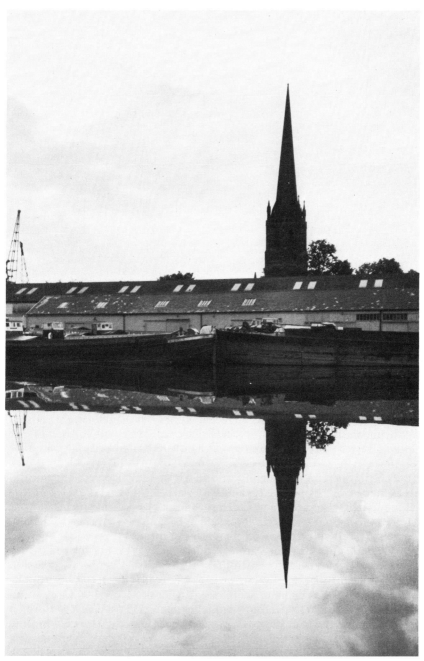

Goole

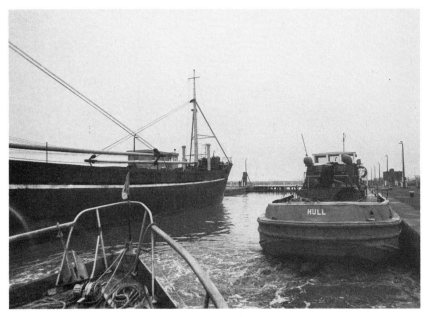

Ocean Lock, Goole: a unique experience connecting the Yorkshire Ouse and the canal navigation.

much worse than they are, for there are many good men and true who will help cruising folk through, thus reducing any chance of it being an ordeal by water. There is a harbour radio station that will also go out of its way to help you; that is, if you keep your traffic to the proper channels, at the proper times and in the proper manner. The locks are generally very busy, and leisure craft are, quite understandably, asked to accept that precedence will be given to commercial vessels. There are three entrance locks as described in the paragraphs on Goole in the section on the Ouse: Ocean, Ouse and Victoria. Ocean Lock is probably the best known and busiest, and it is a piece of incredible engineering at 24 metres wide by 110 metres long with water depths over the sill of 6 metres at mean high water neaps and 8 metres at mean high water springs. And once inside, this locked commercial lake seems to go on for ever in almost every direction – veritably a port-within-a-port. For details see page 186.

Moving inland along the Aire & Calder, the first part of the route out of Goole is busy with barge traffic from the BWB and the commercial operators, and the outskirts right up to the bridge at Rawcliffe are scenically grim and uncared for. But, in common with later stretches on the way to Castleford, it is being improved at its banksides with dredging, piling and near-landscaping by BWB. This is a popular spot for cruising folk from the area because of the nearby pub. Maximum draught to get in to the side without benefit of ladder or plank is about 4'6", but if you are able to choose your spot, you may find the odd hole with a little more. If you are getting near the 6' mark, then it is best to hope to find some co-operative skipper of a shallower draught vessel who will welcome you alongside. (In the regular sea-going ports, I have always found that skippers are more than willing to welcome you to share their lines if there is in any way a shortage of berthing space, but the same courtesies do not seem to apply on those inland waterways that are so much further from the sea. Perhaps it is because there is no external threat big enough to bring boaters together in the way that there is when the sea itself can be heard often battering its way through the harbour.)

The first signs of open pleasantness are to be found after the next stretch and on towards the Southfield reservoir and the New Junction Canal (see pp.118-122). Also, on this patch, you are likely to come across vessels with those wheelhouses that lower to go under bridges; they certainly are a sight to make one ponder. It was also in this area that I encountered a matchless skipper who was to become a regular acquaintance of mine. I was monitoring the radio traffic on the Marine band VHF and heard one skipper complaining to the other that he had been at work since five that morning and had not had a cigarette because he had forgotten the wherewithal with which to light one. It was then about nine o'clock. A few minutes later I saw the self-same vessel approaching me through what was still the early morning mist, but the name was painted clearly on the bows and I recognised it from the radio traffic. She was doing a goodly rate of knots, so I shouted him up on the radio and said that if he would slow down as we passed I would throw him a box of *vestas* (or Lucifers, according to your religious preferences). He did so; and on every occasion after that when we passed he would rush to the bows of his vessel furiously miming the

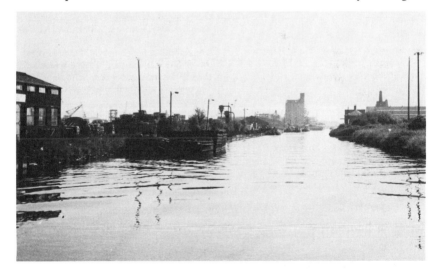

On the way out of Goole, (there is a pleasant lay-by, giving excellent access to the town's facilities – which are something quite else – and providing full maintenance service . . .) and the start of the long haul to Leeds and Wakefield.

striking of a match complete with great grins and thumbs up. His was a shining (or should it be striking?) example of the kind of behaviour that is almost commonplace among the commercial skippers using the Aire & Calder and associated routes. Almost without exception, they are courteous in the extreme to any cruising vessel that shows the least sign of canal sense. One of them even went out of his way to lead me through a thick fog and warn me over the radio of approaching hazards.

The first lock that you meet comes after passing the New Junction. It is Pollington, one of the largest on the navigation and is to be noted specially for the unexpected basin that comes in the middle of the pen. There is nothing for the cruising man immediately by the lock or the banks, though the tiny village of Pollington itself is no more than half a mile away. What is of great interest is to come shortly with the village, basin and club at Heck; and, by heck, not only is there Heck, but also is there Great Heck and Little Heck. This must be an obligatory stop on your itinerary: it is unique.

POLLINGTON LOCK

The Lock,
Pollington,
Goole,
North Humberside
VHF channels 16 and 74

Restricting dimensions 483' x 22' x 9'5"
Rise and fall 7'
Mechanised •
Keeper operated •
Facilities nearby

⚓ WC

📖 George & Dragon, Kings Head –
   approx ½ mile
S General store ½ mile
✉ ½ mile
⚓ Lock tail or Pollington bridge 200 yards
♪ ½ mile

Remarks
Opening times:
Monday-Thursday 0600-2200 hours
Friday 0600-2000 hours
Saturday 0700-1200 hours
           1300-1700 hours
Sunday 0900-1200 hours
           1300-1700 hours

HECK & WHITLEY
Goole 12 miles
Castleford 12 miles

Moorings
A word with the lock-keeper at Whitley Bridge should show a pleasantly sheltered berth or two in the cut just by the lock.

Marina
Heck Basin: The South Yorkshire Boat Club. Dependent upon the state of the canal depth of water, craft of up to 6' can negotiate the basin. There is a restriction on craft above 36' and their general limitations are: 36' x 12' x 3'6". There is also a further restriction: No Hire Craft.

The clubhouse telephone is Whitley Bridge (0977) 661312, and they are also connected to the BWB Land Lines – very helpful. There is not a more friendly club to be found for many a knot.

Club
See above.

Facilities
⚓ ✗ 📖 ♪ S ⚓

Remarks
Don't miss out on The Bay Horse Inn at Heck; the landlords, although changing, seem to retain a connection with things maritime. There is also the small community of Eggborough that should be given a visit. Moorings by the bridge are very convenient. The village shop (one of the classic corner shops) must be unique. Do give it your custom if only to taste its other-world character and don't walk into the bedroom or the parlour thinking one of them to be the grocery section.

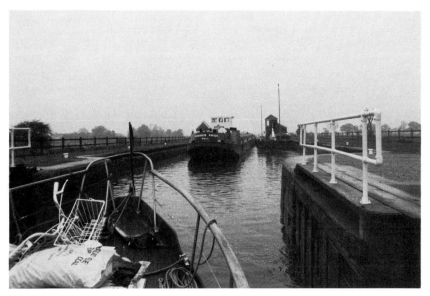

Pollington Lock is an interesting variation upon the usual design, size and shape, with its capacious 'double pound'. It is one of the busiest on the system. In fact, there are three pounds, but BWB are modest about it.

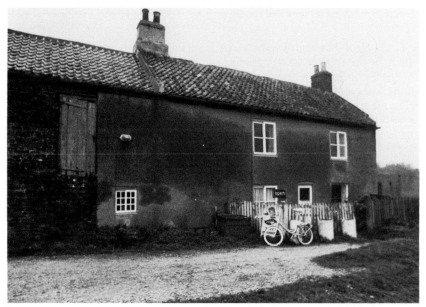

Great Heck is a unique spot; and this is the private house that is the small community's only shop – also unique.

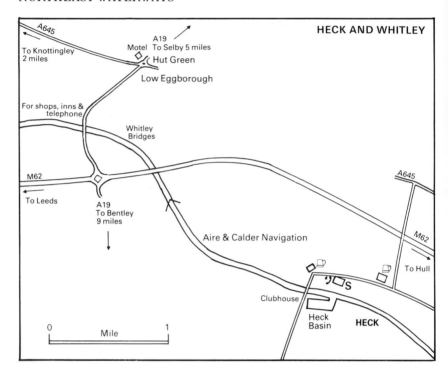

Great Heck lies mid-way between Low Eggborough and Pollington. It is closer to the Aire & Calder Navigation than it is to the M62, although not much; but in any case the slow behemoths of the former and the juggernauts of the latter all leave it in peace. In fact, the only sign of any noisy travel comes from the huge lorries that are working from the local quarry, and, in season, from the sugar beet traffic that hurtles through the village with such regularity that it is virtually a convoy. However, that is for a limited season only: while stocks last. In general though, Heck's stock (that is, standing) is firmly rooted in sound stock (that is, ancestry) and if anyone were ever to take stock of Heck's standing on the stock exchange they would find its share of the shares to be right at the top with the greatly preferred.

Great Heck is also near Little Heck, and those who live in either Heck or even nearby parts will tend to say: 'We live by Heck'. The *Concise Oxford* is illuminating on the subject: HECK 1. noun: obstruction in the river; 2. noun: euphemism for HELL, especially in imprecations. Thus, there is either way, a strong indication that a visitor should be wary. In fact, there is no need, for the place is at one and the same time so under-visited, under-nourished and under-rated and also left behind to become no more than a tiny ripple in the stream of the 20th century, that an amiable welcome is given to all and sundry . . . and the children still approach strangers in the street.

Indeed, so relaxed, informal and friendly is it that the one village shop is more a home than a house and more both than a business. If you enter, unknowingly and untutored, at a normal pace for an ordinary shop, you will probably propel yourself straight upstairs into private quarters. If you avoid that hazard, you may well get caught by the next: turning the 'wrong' way when inside the entrance; once again you have a pretty good chance of invading private territory. And even when you have found the commercial department, you will need a little time to stand and stare and adjust to the atmosphere, for it is a bit like having a shopful of goodies in your front living room. But trade is trade for a nation of shopkeepers and no matter which generation of the incumbents serves you, you will, more or less, be sure to get what you want.

The only way of telling that the place is a shop, is a small sign near the house that bears the legend, 'Open' – a clear case of open house . . . or is it private shop? Not far away, another kind of house altogether, a public house, stands at the big bend in the road, ready to catch you whether coming or going. It is the Bay Horse Inn where the landlord often exuberantly presides over an establishment that is a standing invitation. Extremes are catered for: you can indulge in a yard of ale (on the stop watch if you want your 'record' time to be enrolled above the bar) or take the smallest of cocktails with the biggest of kicks. But don't expect the landlord always to be in calling distance or even in residence. While individual landlords come and go, there seems to be a continuum of their interest in 'messing about in boats', and it is always possible that urgent matters may have summoned them to the waterway.

Not far from the pub and just over the hardly negotiable bridge is another 'wet' matter: the headquarters of the South Yorkshire Boat Club. (That bridge is not to be dismissed: it must be impossible for two cars to pass in comfort and if a Mini were to meet a sugar beeter, one of them would have to give way!) The club is to be found in the basin that was originally built as a railway terminus for quarried stone onwards to Goole and then to London. Due to an oversight, negotiations with the Aire & Calder management never got off the ground, with the result that it was never put into commission and was allowed to lurk in dereliction until 1968 when it was developed into the yacht haven.

The friendly quiet, but not too quiet, that surrounds this restored pool is symptomatic of the delights that are to be found, largely and generally, in the feet-on-the-ground backwater that makes Great Heck the heck of a great place that it is.

Whitley Lock and the old and new bridges are not far away on the way to Knottingley. Hereabouts are some more neat place names: Low and High Eggborough and Hut Green; and both at the lock and by the bridges there are moorings a'plenty, with facilities of the small village settlement close by – and a pub even closer.

From here on until after Castleford, the scenery is not what is usually known as 'tourist attractive'; but it is well worth concentrating on since it combines some of the best of Yorkshire's open views with some of the most dramatically overpowering sights one could imagine of industrial architectural constructions. There are plenty of facilities at Knottingley, especially pubs and shops,

WHITLEY LOCK

Whitley Lock House,
Whitley Bridge,
Goole,
North Humberside
VHF channels 16 and 74

Restricting dimensions   460' x 22' x 9'3"
Rise and fall   6'
Mechanised   ●
Keeper operated   ●

Facilities nearby
⚓ ◼ Sanitary station
▱ Jolly Miller ¾ mile
S General store ¾ mile
✉ ¾ mile

Remarks
Opening times as for Pollington Lock.

but they are all well away from the canal; and winding its way through this community, the canal will proceed to surprise you with unexpected scenic vistas at bendy spots just where you might meet up with some commercial traffic.

After Knottingley, there is nothing to compete with Ferrybridge; indeed, the place is absolutely *sui generis* and when viewed from the river shows itself off as if it possesses a will of its own. Here, the power stations reach for the sky and the old Great North Road, now the 'new' A1(T), cuts right across the skyline. In times past, Tom Puddings used to serve these stations with coal, but they have now been superseded by the amazing push'n'pull (or push-tow) units of Cawood Hargreaves: those water-horses that manoeuvre their laden floating coal hods to deliver to the power stations. (They really do deserve to be called hippopotami: *hippos* – horse, and *potamos* – river.) But not only do they push'n'pull hereabouts, they also lift'n'drop; and it is a sight not to be missed when the huge tippers go through their motions shifting something like 1000 tons an hour. Nothing can equal the looming stature of the girder work, skeletal and imperative, as it points up and away from the solid curves of the earthbound towers. In centuries gone by, cathedrals were built with spires to aid man to see his way clear to God, if not indeed to ascend them for direct communion. These substitutes, especially when seen in strong silhouette, indicate an entirely different heaven on earth, and are much more to be likened with a Hades or an Inferno. They may seem Titans, or a kind of *deus ex machina*, these heroes who work the mighty plant and two-handed engines that dominate this locality, but I know from the generous help offered to me when *Valcon* was being stubbornly temperamental about something nasty in the gearbox, that there is a heart that beats with compassion yet at the centre of the CH operation. Unlikely as it seems, there are pubs, shops and fish'n'chips nearby and accessible.

To the east end of the vast industrial conurbation that is formed by Knottingley, Ferrybridge, Pontefract and Castleford the Aire & Calder Navigation has its first real business with the River Aire. There is a junction with the cut at Bank Dole that gives on to the river. This, in turn, leads through Beal and Haddlesey to the Selby Canal, and the rest of the unnavigable River Aire as it makes its way to the Yorkshire Ouse. (Selby Canal: pp.174-16.) At the west end of Knottingley and well before the Ferrybridge power stations, the navigation is joined by the river proper, and up to Castleford they share the course. Which no doubt explains the more attractive vistas that are to come.

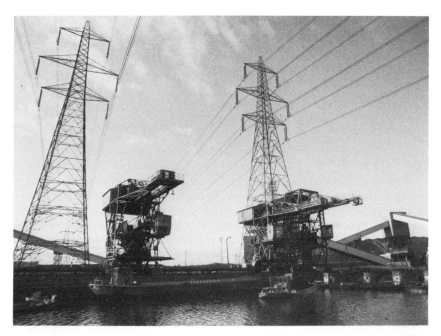

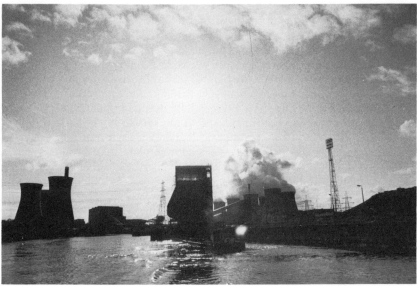

These may not be your actual dark, satanic mills; but there is little here to remind one of England's green and pleasant land. Their aspects continually change and are never less than dramatic; usually they are compelling.

FERRYBRIDGE LOCK

No 2 Lock House,
Ferrybridge,
Knottingley,
West Yorkshire
VHF channels 16 and 74

Restricting dimensions 475' x 25' x 8'6"
Rise and fall Flood lock, open in normal river
conditions.
Mechanised •
Keeper operated •

Facilities nearby
⚓ 🔧 ♨

🏠 Golden Lion, Magnet Inn – 100 yards.
S General stores, newsagents, fish shop, etc.
✉ 100 yards
☎ 100 yards

Remarks
Opening times as for Pollington Lock.
The Golden Lion public house has full hotel
facilities plus lunch and evening meals.

After the drama of the apparently never-ending line of the Ferrybridge
power stations, there is a change from 200 ton barges being lifted vertiginously
in their entirety and there comes a break for light and relief as Brotherton
comes into view. For a while the scenery is unbroken and good to behold, and
the feeling of the waterway is one of calm. Here you should bring your eyes
down from any soul-searching, heavenward glances that might have been
inspired by 'that sweet city with her dreaming spires' (if Ferrybridge may be
permitted the accolade of Oxford's gown), to concentrate on the banks just
above water level especially those to the north. Here are to be seen glorious
combinations and permutations of shades of red, yellow, orange, blue and
brown; and, in addition, there will be an extremely frothy wake to mark your
progress (probably undesirable to conservationists, but very pretty to contemplate) and perhaps urge towards Bulhome Lock, which tells that
Castleford is not far away.

Apart from the usual problems of not finding sufficient water near the banks
where there are supposed to be places 'set aside' for mooring, I can find not a
word of criticism to offer about Castleford. Just by the road bridge of the A656,
the old Roman Road, is an excellent spot to moor; and there are usually a few
'retired' barges permitting an outside berth for deeper draught boats. Close by
there are two pubs: the Griffin and the Volunteer. In my opinion, they are
quite different and in two separate worlds, perhaps even mutually exclusive
ones. I am sure it will not take the dedicated reader long to determine which is
the favoured one, for while both houses have character and characters, only
one of them did I find in any way appealing.

Almost next door is an auto-spares shop that is pretty special in that its
atmosphere is more akin to a social organisation than a business one; but there
is nothing at all unbusinesslike about the actual service, advice or stocks – and
in particular it is a great joy in this man's world of motors, engines and bikes
to be attended upon by a woman whose knowledge of the bits and pieces of
automobile engineering would leave a good few male mechanics if not actually
standing, then at least hitching a ride.

Just a little further into town brings you across the bridge and near the market and main shopping area. The market rates as one of the best in the area, and
just across the road there is a first class glazier and merchant in glass.

BULHOLME LOCK

No 1 Bungalow,
Bulholme Lodge,
Lock Lane,
Castleford,
West Yorkshire
VHF channels 16 and 74

Restricting dimensions   462'-1320' x 22'
Rise and fall   7'
Mechanised   •
Keeper operated   •
Facilities nearby

   ▭ Old Mill and Griffin approx ½ mile
   S ½ mile
   ⚓ ⊠ Lock Lane ½ mile

Remarks
Opening times:
Monday-Thursday 0700-1730 hours
Friday 0700-1630 hours
Saturday 0700-1200 hours
          1300-1700 hours
Sunday 0900-1200 hours
       1300-1700 hours

CASTLEFORD JUNCTION LOCK

5, Junction Houses,
Castleford,
West Yorkshire
VHF channels 16 and 74

Restricting dimensions   22' between the gates
Rise and fall   Flood Lock
Mechanised   •
Keeper operated   •
Facilities nearby

   🐟 Local garage
   ▭ Griffin and Old Mill 200 yards
     Grocery ½ mile
   ⊠ ½ mile
     Overnight only
   🔧 1 miles

Remarks
See Bulhome Lock for opening times.

CASTLEFORD

Goole 24 miles
Leeds 10 miles
Wakefield 7 miles

Moorings
BWB moorings in the bight.

Boatyard
There is no boatyard; but there are mechanics,
engineers and garages in the town. There is an
auto-spares shop by the bridge. Cawood-
Hargreaves Engineering repair depot is also
close by on the canal.

Facilities
🐟 ✕ 🔧 ▭ ⊠ 🏪

Most other facilities can be found in the town,
after a bit of a search.

Remarks
Although Castleford is not what you would call
a 'natural' for a boating centre; I find it a place
of considerable appeal with as many domestic
and social facilities as you could want . . . and,
with a bit of searching around and string pulling here and there, you should be able to get all
the maintenance work you might need on a
cruise attended to. If not, there is always the
boatyard of Harkers at Knottingley.

Castleford is also the headquarters of the engineering section of Cawood Hargreaves, so there is always a good bit of their traffic moving around and about but it is in a wide stretch of the canal and they are always sensible of the needs of responsible boaters. And here too, by the lock just before the junction of the Rivers Aire and Calder, is the headquarters of the Castleford section of the British Waterways Board and even they have no landscaped lock or basin to view from their offices. It is all, you might say, satisfactory; but on the optimistic front it is at least functional, efficient and tidy. I allowed myself an extra-special peek at the typists and secretaries in the BWB offices because of the local ditty that claims 'All the girls are so fair, 'cos they wash in the Calder and bathe in the Aire.'

There are overnight moorings in the bight, with bollards and rings. There is also a BWB sanitary station, water, toilet and rubbish disposal. Many people find it worth staying for a while just to get photographs of commercial boats negotiating the bend and the lock entrance. There is a gantry by the lock-keeper's office and this provides an excellent vantage point; he should, of course, be approached for his permission. Do not moor alongside the wall on the right outside the lock between the junction and the old Allerton coal staithes. Apart from passing commercial traffic and the attendant dangers, the area has been, unhappily, notorious for vandals, in particular for boats being cast adrift. One such, the *Thomas*, is still wrecked across Castleford weir. There is a pub alongside the high wall, but you should keep your eye on your boat; and it is best to use rings, taking your lines back to the boat, not just pins. It is worth a reminder here that it is never sensible to tie up on a main line stretch. Passing commercial traffic, which starts at 0600, and sometimes before, will pull out pins and even stout land anchors with little difficulty.

After Castleford Lock (in fact, before it even, for the keeper will demand to know) the first decision is whether to turn to the right for the River Aire and all stations to Leeds, or to forge straight ahead on the River Calder and to make for Wakefield. We shall take the Leeds line first.

Castleford to Leeds

It is only ten miles from Castleford junction to Leeds and since there are only seven locks, it takes no time at all to make the trip. Another reason why it is such a smoothly swift leg is that the lock-keepers are all extremely efficient and keen to see you through with as much speed and ease as they can promote. There is also little to tempt the waterborne traveller to stay his heart, mind or boat; indeed, the only place that I recommend for a proper visit is Woodlesford. Otherwise it is big locks and fairly depressing surroundings all the way into Leeds City Basin. There are many potentially interesting locations and buildings on the way that could be put into order and improve the amenities and aesthetics for townies, rustics as well as caravanners and boaters. There are however two places of interest: one a village, Woodlesford; and the other a museum, Thwaites Mill. The museum is worth an exploratory perambulation

KIPPAX LOCK

Kippax Lock House,
Methley,
Leeds

Restricting dimensions   227′9″ x 23′6″
Rise and fall   7′6″
Mechanised   •
Keeper operated   •
Facilities nearby
⚓

🍴 Commercial Inn 1 mile
S General Stores 1½ miles
✉ Approximately 1½ miles
♪ Approximately 1½ miles

Remarks
Opening times as for Bulholme Lock.

LEMONROYD LOCK

Lemonroyd Lock House,
Methley,
Leeds

Restricting dimensions   257′ x 23′
Rise and fall   6′6″
Mechanised   •
Keeper operated   •
Facilities nearby
⚓

🍴 United Kingdom, Royal Oak – 10 minutes
walk.

Remarks
Opening times as for Bulholme Lock.

WOODLESFORD LOCK

Woodlesford Lock House,
Woodlesford,
Leeds

Restricting dimensions   257′ x 23′
Rise and fall   9′
Mechanised   •
Keeper operated   •
Facilities nearby
⚓ ⚓

wc But belongs to lock-keeper's cabin
🍴 500 yards
🍴 Two Pointers and White Hart
(caters for children) approx   700 yards
S Supermarket, newsagents, fish shop,
bakery approx. 700 yards
✉ Approx. 700 yards
♪ 700 yards from lock

Remarks
Opening times as for Bulholme Lock.
One of the pleasantest locks on the navigation.
Good facilities and also there is Bingo 800 yards
from lock! Most boat people try to make it to
this lock to moor craft.

while the village is worth a perambulatory exploration; both can be taken in depth, but one will take just that much longer than the other. Woodlesford calls first.

Although the scenery just manages to suggest that you are in the heart of the country, there is quite a lot of commercial traffic using this stretch. It is therefore not only courteous but also sensible and safety conscious to ask the lock-keeper for his permission and advice about where to berth, especially if overnight.

Once upon a time, in the village of Woodlesford, some years ago, there lived a certain Mr. B. He was a great benefactor of the church, so, in his honour, they called the main street, Church Street.

Once upon a time, some different years ago, there lived a different Mr. B. He was a great benefactor of the chapel, so, in his honour, they called the main street, Chapel Street.

Nowadays, the honours seem about equal; or if they aren't the Woodlesfordites are hedging their bets, for everyone told me it is now called High Street. High it certainly is, perched on top of a steep hill that leads down to a ravine, a minor back road, a river (the Aire), a canal (the Aire & Calder), and finally gives access to the nearby A624, the M62, the M1 and is no distance at all from Temple Newsham and Rothwell where there must be the oldest surviving iron-mongers from the pages of Dickens.

There are four unusual and striking factors about Woodlesford. First, start-ing at water level, there is a lock that affords the prettiest and most convenient stopping off place between Leeds and the Humber. It is well kept by a devotee of patience and crossword puzzles and shows weeping willows by a small drive to the water's edge. It is close to the river, which at that point is almost ruggedly craggy and almost abandoned.

The view is dominated by Whitbread's brewery chimney. Sad to say this is now not a brewery at all, but it used to be. In its glory it was Bentley's York-shire Brewery and was founded as the Eshald Well Brewery in 1828 and writ-ten up in the *Licensed Victuallers' Guardian* in 1857 as follows: 'It is well known that the natural springs which abound in Leeds and its vicinity contain two ingredients which especially adapt it to brewing purposes.' For those who care about these things, they are rich in carbonate and sulphate of lime. For my part, the waters as they flow in those parts show no sign of being natural nor of being suitable for consumption. Although it is no longer a brewery, it is still a working drinks establishment and its main entrance, walls, arches and nearby attached cottages are all well preserved, in fact as well as by order.

Closer to the village from the lock comes an unexpected oasis of contempor-ary houses and gardens. They, like the equally unexpected modern shopping precinct in the heart of Old Woodlesford, are the brain child of one Leslie Appleyard of E. Appleyard Limited; and they hope in the future to expand their riverside development and then to provide a small basin for narrow boats and cruisers.

One householder in this stately estate was in fact so pleased with the design that he bought two to use as one; so his family had two of everything and perhaps even more. He was not entirely content with Woodlesford as it had grown. 'It has changed for the better, and for the worse. There are more amenities, but the great British heritage and village traditions of caring and considering for one another have gone.'

Back at the top of the hill, past the newsagents where they bake in the back so that your glasses will steam up and prevent you from getting a free look at the day's papers, there is an intriguing contiguity: next to the Old Church stands the New House. Built mainly in slate and glass, it resembles a modern interpretation of an American Indian tepee. Local legend is by no means in unison about the amazing glazing: I was told it was 'solo' heating; 'solar' heat-ing; a solarium; an experimental conservatory; and 'just some extra storage space they don't know what to do with.'

Leslie Appleyard is of the opinion that when that house and his estate development came about in the 60s or so, 'planning was in a more informal, creative and imaginative stage and you could get on with things that were exciting and worthwhile.'

Fortunately for everyone, Woodlesford now contains the best of the past (for its many really old cottages are being pleasingly renovated); the best of the present (for all the development does nothing but enhance the neighbourhood); and its future must surely be promising for all.

The lock-keeper himself is a friendly, patient man who could not be more helpful; and he has made his patch something of an attractive oasis. I can vividly remember the first time I stayed there: it was in December; a bleak month after a particularly harsh autumn's cruising, and I counted myself fortunate that I had discovered a positive sanctuary. I was called on by all kinds of visitors and friendly neighbours including the police, who told me such a gripping tale of riverside suicide and life or death endeavours that I completely forgot the domestic chores I was supposed to be attending to. The result was a bilge filled with overflown water from the hose and a small fire by the stove where I was airing my recently washed socks. My coal supplies were delivered on to the deck at a better price than I had had to pay when humping them home myself; and the passing barge skippers could not have been more considerate in their manoeuvres in and out of the lock and always had a word and a wave.

True, the main part of the village is at the top of a very steep climb from the lock, but once you are there you will never question the expenditure of effort for there is everything there a boating man might want (and quite a few most boaters would never think of): from an acupuncturist, a baker and a chapman or colporteur to xenophiles and xenophobes, yobs (for sadly, vandalism is rife in the village, but not down by the lock) and zealots. Woodlesford is a place for the connoisseur of idiosyncratic England, and there is no doubt in my mind that it is best visited by boat.

FISHPOND LOCK

Fishpond Lock House,
Bullough Lane,
Rothwell,
Leeds

Restricting dimensions   287' x 12'
Rise and fall   6'6"
Mechanised   ●
Keeper operated   ●
Facilities nearby
🪝 ⚓
Remarks
Opening tims as for Bulholme Lock.

KNOSTROP FALL LOCK

Knostrop Fall Lock House,
Thwaite Gate,
Stourton,
Leeds

Restricting dimensions   216' x 22'
Rise and fall   6'6"
Mechanised   ●
Keeper operated   ●
Facilities nearby
🪝
🛢 Oil and petrol
🍺 Crooked Billet and Punch Clock – 300 yards
✉ 400 yards

Remarks
Opening times as for Bulholme Lock.

LEEDS

Goole 34 miles
Wakefield 17 miles
Castleford 10 miles

Moorings
BWB moorings by City Lock, Leeds Lock and in the basin. Yorkshire Canal Services also provide berthing facilities in the basin.

Marina
There is no marina as such, but the basin does provide some sort of marina facility. It is used mainly, however, as a staging station and not a cruising or leisure base, although there is much to see and to do in the city.

Club
There is no club on site, but there is a waterside café. (The delights of the huge Dragonara are not far away and its tower block cannot be missed. There are also the hazards and delights, if you care for that sort of thing, of the Dark Arches.)

Facilities
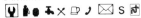

There are resident engineers, electricians and other craftsmen who, by personal arrangement with a skipper, will undertake boat work at the going rate.

Remarks
Leeds has much more to offer from the city point of view than it has as a water base. It is important in so far as it stands at the junction of the Aire & Calder and the Leeds & Liverpool. There is much for a canal enthusiast to lament and even more for a compassionate eye to photograph. But as a holiday base it has not as yet got under way.

LEEDS LOCK

Clarence Road,
Leeds 10

Restricting dimensions This lock is a basin lock (3 sets of gates): Top, middle and low. Low – Middle 153′. Middle – Top 71′ x 18′
Rise and fall 4′
Hand operated •
Boater operated •
Facilities nearby

🛢	Diesel
🖙	½ mile, city centre
S	½ mile, city centre
✉	½ mile, city centre

Remarks
Open at all times.

The other calling off spot is the industrial museum run by the Thwaites Mill Society. There is a pleasant jetty just before the bridge, and while the environs leave much to be desired, the frontage of the project from the river is beginning to grow in appeal. And then from here on it is a long, slow haul into the centre of Leeds where, once installed in the basin, you can choose between the Dark Arches, which really are still very dark indeed, and the bright lights of the Dragonara hotel and gaming club. It is a shame that there is still so much to be done to put this area to rights. The immediate environs and also the periphery of the canal area are in a parlous state, and while there are plans afoot the present reality is one of dismal decay.

The first time I approached City Lock my eye was caught by a photographer and his model who were doing their best to find a canalside location that did not feature half-sinking boats or degraded fabrics. My immediate impression was one of doom and gloom, and nothing that I have experienced since suggests that the place is getting its fair share of care and attention, if not indeed protection. If ever there was a spot that justified the skipper going ahead by road to check out the arrangements, this must be it. The river section must be seen to be believed, and I feel no inclination whatsoever to proceed much further than City Lock; and in the past I have always retreated to the lotus eaters' paradise at Woodlesford.

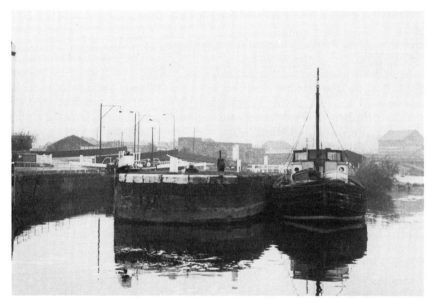

All roads lead to Rome – all roads roam to Leeds: the veritable end of the Aire & Calder Navigation, where, after Leeds Canal Basin, the waterway becomes the Leeds & Liverpool.

Castleford to Wakefield

It is not far from Castleford Junction to Wakefield Ings Lock, a short seven miles. (And before too many readers launch diatribes at me because they prefer Ing to Ings, let me state that I have spent hours on research on this particular, and the best authority I can find adjudicates in favour of the plural. In any case, that is how the Ordnance Survey pundits refer to it.) The exit from Castleford is straight ahead out of the lock, having checked with the keeper and followed his signals.

Perhaps this is a good place to remind readers that all locks on this system are controlled by traffic lights, which are in turn controlled by lock-keepers. This qualification is an important one, since you may well find that the gates are open and the lights are at red but there is a keeper waving you in by hand. In principle, it makes a neat point for debate as to who or what should be obeyed; but in practice I always respond to the latest signal that I have been given and in these cases it means doing what the keeper wants. There is also another point worth noting, and this applied particularly to the Wakefield Arm, and that is that all locks have been enlarged at some time or another but their doors, paddles or cloughs have been left in their original positions. This means that water will come in at about the centre of the lock, and it is a good idea to ask the keeper for advice about where to tie up. He will usually tell you where he would like you to go and that will take care of all problems.

There is not a lot before Stanley Ferry to catch the eye. I have been told that there is often a good supply of farm fresh comestibles available by the lock at Birkwood. Undoubtedly there is much of interest at Stanley Ferry where you can see aqueducts both ancient and modern. The new version, no doubt much safer and more substantial than the older one, cannot rival it when it comes to aesthetics, for the original is in the style of the famous bridge at Sydney, Australia. There is a thriving community here, part commercial/industrial thanks to the British Waterways Board engineering yard where once were built Tom Puddings, and part bucolic/rural with a museum piece of a swing bridge (Ramsden's). Here it is possible to tie up alongside the north bank and take the short walk up an unmade-up, mainly unlit road to the main road and its nearby Ship Inn. You will find that the landlord is likely to give you a special welcome if he discovers you have come from a boat. Also near here is the former office of the Aire & Calder Navigation Company, which is now in a state of dereliction, in spite of attempts by devotees to have it converted into an information centre. Bartholomew's grave is to be found in Stanley churchyard up the hill.

WOODNOOK LOCK

Foxholes Lane,
Altofts,
Normanton,
West Yorkshire

Restricting dimensions   214'6" x 18'6"
Rise and fall   11'6"
Mechanised   •
Keeper operated   •
Facilities nearby
⚓

Remarks
Opening times as for Bulholme Lock.

KINGS ROAD LOCK

Foxholes Lane,
Altofts,
Normanton,
West Yorkshire

Restricting dimensions   215'6" x 18'6"
Rise and fall   6'6"
Mechanised   •
Keeper operated   •
Facilities nearby
⚓ ⬓
Miners Arms, Poplar, Horse & Jockey, ¾ mile
General stores, newspapers, etc. approx. ½ mile

✉ ¾ mile

Remarks
Opening times as for Bulholme Lock.

BIRKWOOD LOCK

Altofts,
Normanton,
West Yorkshire

Restricting dimensions   214' x 22'6"
Rise and fall   6'6"
Mechanised   •
Keeper operated   •
Facilities nearby
None
Remarks
Opening times as for Bulholme Lock.

RAMSDEN'S SWING BRIDGE

Ward Lane,
Stanley,
Wakefield,
West Yorkshire

Restricting dimensions   21' wide
Hand operated   •
Keeper operated   •
Facilities nearby
⚓
⬓ Ship Inn – ¼ mile
S Newsagent and off-licence approx. ½ mile
✉ 1 mile
☎ ½ mile

Remarks
Opening times as for Bulholme Lock.
Moorings on bank towards aqueduct dangerous dues to tankers making wide sweep out of aqueduct.

BROADREACH FLOOD LOCK

Broadreach Lock House,
Linton Road,
Park Lodge Lane,
Wakefield,
West Yorkshire

Restricting dimensions   465' x 18' x 6'
Rise and fall   See *Remarks*
Hand operated   •
Boater operated   •
If lock-keeper is not present. Gates and clough gear to be left exactly as found. If clough gear slightly raised leave it the same degree open to maintain feed.

Facilities nearby

Remarks
Opening times as for Bulholme Lock. Broadreach is a flood lock, therefore, rise and fall governed by flood water, otherwise canal and river are the same level.

FALL INGS LOCK

Doncaster Road,
Wakefield,
West Yorkshire

Restricting dimensions   128' x 17' x 6'
Rise and fall   9'6"
Hand operated   •
Boater operated   •
Windlass required   •
Facilities nearby

⚓

🛢 Oil, petrol – 200 yards
🏪 Several – 200 yards
Newsagents, take-away fish and chips, etc.
☏ 600 yards

From here there is little of note until the lock just outside Wakefield, the one I have already referred to 'Fall Ings. It certainly is 'Fall Ing' into such disrepair that it will surely next 'Fall Into' disrepute. British Waterways still post a notice requesting users to close all gates before leaving the lock, in spite of the fact that it is physically impossible to comply with the request because of the configuration of wind, water and gravity and the state of disrepair of the apparatus. Needless to say, I, naïvely overconscientious as ever, struggled through four attempts at obeying the decree before coming to the conclusion that I was succeeding in nothing more than tilting at lock gates that would never be less than malevolent.

Such an uninviting initiation ceremony into the waters of the Calder & Hebble at Wakefield is discouraging; but it is misleadingly so, for the lock stands guardian to a basin, canal and river stretch within the town that is not only central (and there are plenty of facilities: domestic, social and boating) but also pretty to look at from land or water with some attractive, mature trees and a very reasonably kept weir. Wakefield itself is a bit of a Janus, since looking one way it is part of the Aire & Calder and looking the other it is part of the Calder & Hebble. Either way, it is both beginning and end of both systems, and as such is undoubtedly worth a visit.

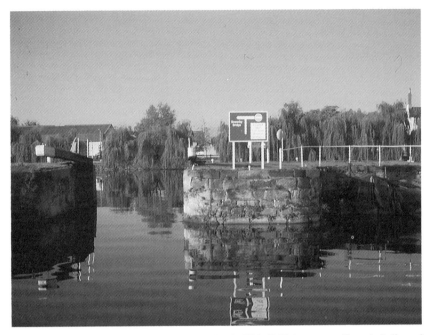

Once through the challenge offered by Fall Ings Lock, Wakefield shows a scruffy underbelly and then blossoms into a quite beautiful experience as the river joins the environs of the town. The centre (and also the weir) are to the right.

The Calder & Hebble Navigation

The Calder & Hebble, like the Aire & Calder, is a river navigation with canal sections. Wherever there is a canal section there is also an unguarded weir and special flood gates at the upstream end. The navigation should be tackled as if it were a full-blown river navigation; and passages should not be undertaken in flood conditions. On such waterways, it is always advisable for buoyancy aids to be worn. The BWB staff close the flood gates whenever their 'safety' levels are reached.

Different from the Aire & Calder, indeed, from all the other canal sections in this volume, the Calder & Hebble has a system of working its paddles that requires a special staff, the famous 'handspike': a length of hardwood about 3′ x 2″ x 3″. On occasions, one such is to be found chained to the lock, but it is best to carry your own on board. They can be purchased through the usual channels.

The main places of note are Horbury, Thornhill, Dewsbury, Mirfield, Huddersfield, Halifax and Sowerby Bridge; and in its 21 miles it winds its way through some of our classic industrial building examples, as well as some extraordinarily beautiful stretches of country in its upper reaches.

DISTANCES IN MILES
Main Line

Sowerby Bridge	Salterhebble	Elland Wharf	Elland Low Lock	Brighouse Wharf	Cooper Bridge	Shepley Bridge	Calder Wharf	Double Locks	Horbury Bridge	Wakefield
2.3										
3.5	1.2									
4.0	1.7	0.5								
6.5	4.2	3.0	2.5							
9.2	6.9	5.7	5.2	2.7						
12.0	9.7	8.5	8.0	5.5	2.8					
13.1	10.8	9.6	9.1	6.6	3.9	1.1				
14.5	12.2	11.0	10.5	8.0	5.3	2.5	1.4			
16.8	14.5	13.3	12.8	10.3	7.6	4.8	3.7	2.3		
21.5	19.2	18.0	17.5	15.0	12.3	9.5	8.4	7.0	4.7	

Maximum Size of Craft

Section	Length	Beam	Draught	Headroom
Aire & Calder Navigation (Fall Ings Lock) to below Broad Cut Upper Lock	120'0"	18'0"	6'6"	11'7"
Broad Cut Upper Lock to below Mill Bank Lock	65'0"	17'6"	6'0"	10'3"
Mill Bank Lock to below Long Cut End Flood Lock	57'6"	14'2"	5'7"	10'3"
Long Cut End Flood Lock to below Brighouse Low Lock	57'6"	14'2"	5'4"	10'3"
Brighouse Low Lock to Sowerby Bridge	57'6"	14'2"	5'0"	9'3"
Dewsbury Branch	57'6"	14'1"	5'0"	8'0"
Huddersfield Broad Canal	57'6"	14'2"	4'6"	8'9"

WAKEFIELD TO SOWERBY

Moorings

This stretch of waterway is extremely well served with domestic, social and boating facilities. There are mooring and boatyard amenities at the following places:

West Riding Marine, Thornes Wharf, Wakefield ☎ (0924) 377676

Mirfield Boatyard, Ledgard Bridge Dockyard, Mirfield ☎ (0924) 492007

Robinson Hire Cruisers, Savile Town Wharf, Dewsbury ☎ (0924) 467976

Aspley Wharf Marina, Aspley Basin, Huddersfield ☎ (0484) 514123

Brighouse Marine, Wharf Street, Brighouse ☎ (0484) 721867

Sowerby Marina, The Wharf, Sowerby Bridge ☎ (0422) 832922

There are also sanitary station facilities at the following BWB stations: Wakefield Flood Lock; Shipley Bridge; Brighouse Basin; Sowerby Bridge and Salterhebble.

Facilities

If these are not always immediately to hand, you can rest assured that they are not far away.

Remarks

This is probably one of the most favoured stretches, containing some of the greatest contrasts and some of the best joys of canal life; especially for narrow boat enthusiasts, although there is always a welcome place for all GRP cruisers.

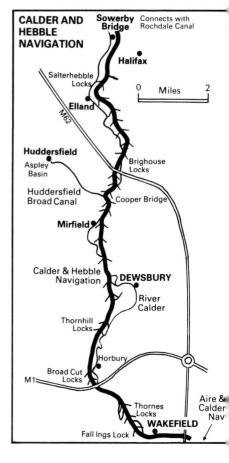

There are many remains of the original route to be found on the canal. For example, the Navigation public house at Broad Cut faces the 'wrong' way. At first, the canal passed by its front door, but when a new cut was made to bypass some difficult river sections, the front door became the back one. I have it on really excellent authoritative recommendation that the Tetley's bitter here, drawn by Frank from the wood, is 'nectar'.

At Horbury bridge, the first arch of the present road bridge is in fact a canal arch. The navigation used to run on the north side of the river forming an island between the river and the canal. A name plate still says *The Island* and there is a Ship Inn at quite a distance removed from the present navigation. Before reaching Horbury there is, in a privately owned field, a complete and undamaged lock chamber without gates. It used to lead into the river. At Figure of Three you will see the two present locks, and above them, the remains of a third lock now converted into a bywash. Cold logic would suggest

WAKEFIELD FLOOD LOCK

Barnsley Road,
Wakefield,
West Yorkshire

Restricting dimensions 132' x 19'
Rise and fall River lock only used in flood
Hand operated •
Boater operated •
Windlass required •
Facilities nearby

⚓
🛒 wc 🚽

🏠 ● Oil, petrol, bottle gas – ½ mile
ℭ Thornes Lane – ½ mile

Remarks
Note historic Chantry bridge and chapel, city
centre, Wakefield cathedral, museum
Market: Monday, Friday and Saturday.

THORNES LOCKS

Denby Dale Road,
Wakefield,
West Yorkshire

Restricting dimensions 65' x 14'
Rise and fall 6'6"
Hand operated •
Boater operated •
Windlass required •
Handspike required •
Facilities nearby None

THORNES FLOOD LOCK

Lupset,
Wakefield,
West Yorkshire

Restricting dimensions 71' x 19'6"
Rise and fall River levels – flood lock
Hand operated •
Boater operated •
Windlass required •
Facilities nearby None

BROAD CUT LOW LOCK

Calder Grove,
Wakefield,
West Yorkshire
☎ Wakefield (0924) 272022

Restricting dimensions 65'6" x 17'6"
Rise and fall 9'
Hand operated •
Boater operated •
Windlass required •
Facilities nearby
⚓ 🛒

ℙ Navigation – 200 yards
S Newsagents and general store – ½ mile
✉ ½ mile to main road
ℭ ½ mile to main road

BROAD CUT TOP LOCK

Broadcut Road,
Durkar,
Wakefield,
West Yorkshire

Restricting dimensions 67' x 17'6'
Rise and fall 6'
Hand operated •
Boater operated •
Windlass required •
Facilities nearby

🏠 ½ mile to main road
ℙ Navigation – 400 yards
S General store ½ mile
✉ ½ mile to main road
⚓ Downstream of lock
ℭ ½ mile to main road

FIGURE OF THREE LOCKS

Mitchell Laithes,
Thornhill,
Dewsbury,
West Yorkshire

Restricting dimensions 68' x 17'6"
Rise and fall Top Lock 7'6". Bottom Lock 6'
Hand operated •
Boater operated •
Windlass required •
Handspike required •
Facilities nearby
🛒

that $2 + 1 = 3$; but I am told that that is just rubbish and all those who favour the idea should be examined for faulty brainwork. The 'real' reason is that the twists and turns in the river at that point make a configuration that appears to be a perfect figure '3'.

Next there is the short Dewsbury Arm, home of Robinsons Hire Cruisers. At one time, what is now the Dewsbury Arm was the main line continuing through to rejoin the river at Dewsbury. Then for a period of 21 years, the Calder & Hebble was leased by the Aire & Calder Company who carried out improvements. When the new cut was made from Broad Cut to Thornhill Flood Lock the Dewsbury line was not used. When the Calder & Hebble regained their ownership, they closed the line, sold the land back to the original owners, Savile Estates, and the top section was filled in and built over. The Aire & Calder Co., referred to by my informant as 'crafty devils', saw the potential of their having a base there and secretly bought the lower length from Savile Estates. They then built a warehouse there and extended the basin to its present size. There used to be a fine wooden warehouse there, but it has been put down by BWB. After building a new road and roadbridge from Dewsbury, the Aire & Calder Co. had a neat operational base right in the centre of 'enemy' territory. The Dewsbury Arm is now being improved, mainly after pressure and/or encouragement from the Calder Navigation Society.

MILLBANK LOCK

Thornhill,
Dewsbury,
West Yorkshire

Restricting dimensions 61' x 14'
Rise and fall Approx. 7'6"
Hand operated •
Boater operated •
Windlass required •
Handspike required •
Facilities nearby None

THORNHILL FLOOD LOCK

Thornhill,
Dewsbury,
West Yorkshire

Restricting dimensions 24' x 14'(not operational until further notice)
Rise and fall River lock only used in flood
Hand operated •
Boater operated •
Windlass required •
Facilities nearby None

DOUBLE LOCKS

Lock Street,
Savile Town,
Dewsbury,
West Yorkshire

Restricting dimensions Top Lock 59' x 14'
Low Lock 60' x 14'4"
Rise and fall Top Lock 6'
Low Lock 3'9"
Hand operated •
Boater operated •
Windlass required •
Handspike required •
Facilities nearby ⚓

GREENWOOD LOCK

Fir Cottage,
Shepley Bridge,
Mirfield,
West Yorkshire

Restricting dimensions 81' x 14'
Rise and fall 7'6"
Hand operated •
Boater operated •
Windlass required •
Handspike required •
Facilities nearby None

GREENWOOD FLOOD LOCK

Fir Cottage,
Shepley Bridge,
Mirfield,
West Yorkshire

Restricting dimensions   13'6" Flood gate only
Rise and fall   River levels
Hand operated   •
Boater operated   •
Windlass required   •
Facilities nearby

🍴 Bull (mid-day bar meals), White Swan.
Ship – all ¼ mile away

LEDGARD BRIDGE FLOOD LOCK

Newgate,
Mirfield,
West Yorkshire

Restricting dimensions   148'6" x 13'9"
Rise and fall   Flood lock
Hand operated   •
Boater operated   •
Windlass required   •
Facilities nearby
⚓

🅿 Central garage – ¼ mile
🍴 Approx. ¼ mile away
S Everything you require
✉ ¼ mile
�’

BATTYE CUT LOCK

Battyford,
Mirfield,
West Yorkshire

Restricting dimensions   81' x 13'8"
Rise and fall   9'9"
Hand operated   •
Boater operated   •
Windlass required   •
Facilities nearby
🍴
Pear Tree – ½ mile

BATTYE FLOOD LOCK

Battyford,
Mirfield,
West Yorkshire

Restricting dimensions   13'6" wide
Rise and fall   Flood gates only
Hand operated   •
Boater operated   •
Windlass required   •
Facilities nearby None

Officially the Calder & Hebble from Wakefield to Greenwood Lock is still classified as commercial and, until a few years ago, coal was carried to the now defunct Thornhill power station. The Mirfield Boatyard was formerly Hargreaves, and wooden barges were built and repaired there until steel ones replaced them. Calder & Hebble boats are called 'West Country', and although the derivation is geographical, it has nothing to do with Devon and Cornwall. The explanation is: from the east is the Humber, then the Ouse, then the Aire & Calder, and finally, further west, is the Calder & Hebble. Its locks, once past Broad Cut, were not lengthened; the maximum length of broad boats was restricted to 57'6"; hence 'West Country'. This meant that boats coming from the Rochdale canal at Sowerby Bridge and the Huddersfield Canal at Huddersfield had to tranship.

Above Brighouse, the Calder & Hebble becomes 'pure' canal. However, it was not always so and at Tag Cut there was a lock leading to the river and then coming back in at Elland and so on in loops to Salterhebble where at Hebblemouth it became 'pure' canal to Sowerby Bridge. It is asserted, though

SHEPLEY BRIDGE LOCK

Shepley Bridge,
Mirfield,
West Yorkshire

Restricting dimensions   59' x 14'
Rise and fall   8'6"
Hand operated   •
Boater operated   •
Windlass required   •
Handspike required   •
Facilities nearby
⚓ ⛽ 🚽 Sanitary Station
🗄
White Swan, the Ship (bar meals) – ¼ mile

COOPER BRIDGE LOCK

Bradley,
Huddersfield,
West Yorkshire

Restricting dimensions   60' x 13'6"
Rise and fall   5'6"
Hand operated   •
Boater operated   •
Windlass required   •
Handspike required   •
Facilities nearby
⚓

🛢 Oil, petrol – ½ mile to main road
🗄 Commercial and Three Nuns – ¾ mile
S Butchers and newsagent – ¾ mile
☎ ¾ mile

COOPER BRIDGE FLOOD LOCK

Bradley,
Huddersfield,
West Yorkshire

Restricting dimensions   14'6" wide
Rise and fall   Flood gate only
Hand operated   •
Boater operated   •
Windlass required   •
Facilities nearby
⚓

🛢 Oil, petrol ¼ mile to main road
🗄 Commercial, Three Nuns – ½ mile
S Butchers and newsagents – ¼ mile
☎ ¼ mile up Huddersfield Road

there is little documentation, that it was Brindley who put in a staircase at Salterhebble and this proved to be a failure. Conventional locks were then built but, as traffic could not be interrupted during this building, the new locks were built alongside the old ones; thus accounting for the strange bends in the course of the navigation. The guillotine gate has an interesting background: the road was widened, but someone in authority 'forgot' that the lock gates could not be opened. At Salterhebble the defunct Halifax Arm was built without a natural water supply, so that every drop had to be pumped uphill.

Fans of *The Last of the Summer Wine* will be intrigued to check out some of the locations on the Calder & Hebble; near Kirklees Lock; at Brighouse; and the water-skiing at Cromwell Bottom where the former gravel pit is now a lake. (They might also take a peek at Battye Ford). Sowerby Bridge must be an exciting spot to any canal enthusiast. It was derelict until recently, and after the Calder Navigation Society held a rally there it has become increasingly popular. There are all the amenities that boaters need. The Rochdale Canal is now the subject of restoration, and at Cooper Bridge there is similar betterment going on to improve the Huddersfield Narrow Canal.

KIRKLEES LOW LOCK

Kirklees,
Brighouse,
West Yorkshire

Restricting dimensions   60' x 14'
Rise and fall   8'9"
Hand operated   •
Boater operated   •
Windlass required   •
Handspike required   •
Facilities nearby None

KIRKLEES TOP LOCK

As above

Restricting dimensions   75'9" x 14'
Rise and fall   5'
Hand operated   •
Boater operated   •
Windlass required   •
Handspike required   •
Facilities nearby None

ANCHOR PIT FLOOD LOCK

Brighouse,
West Yorkshire

Restricting dimensions   14'
Rise and fall   River levels – Flood lock
Hand operated   •
Boater operated   •
Windlass required   •
Facilities nearby   ⚓

BRIGHOUSE LOCKS

Mill Lane,
Brighouse,
West Yorkshire

Restricting dimensions   Both locks 61' x 14'
Rise and fall   Bottom 8'. Top 3'6"
Hand operated   •
Boater operated   •
Windlass required   •
Handspike required   •
Facilities nearby
⚓
⚓ ♿ Sanitary Station
🛒 ● Gas, oil, petrol, bottle gas – ¼ mile
⌂ At least 15
S Everything required
✉ ¼ mile to town centre
☎ ¼ mile away

Remarks
Small town with supermarkets; open markets
Wednesday and Saturday all day.

GANNY LOCK

Brighouse,
West Yorkshire

Restricting dimensions   60' x 14'
Rise and fall   10'6"
Hand operated   •
Boater operated   •
Windlass required   •
Facilities nearby

🛒 ½ mile back to Brighouse
⌂ Black Bull
S Brighouse – ¼ mile
✉ Brighouse – ¼ mile
☎ Brighouse – ¼ mile

BROOKFOOT LOCK

Brookfoot,
Brighouse,
West Yorkshire

Restricting dimensions   61' x 14'6"
Rise and fall   5'
Hand operated   •
Boater operated   •
Windlass required   •
Facilities nearby
⌂
Wharf – ½ mile
☎ ½ mile

CROMWELL LOCK

Cromwell Bottom,
Elland,
West Yorkshire

Restricting dimensions   61' x 14'6"
Rise and fall   6'
Hand operated   •
Boater operated   •
Windlass required   •
Handspike required   •
Facilities nearby None

PARK NOOK LOCK

Rawson Pool,
Elland,
West Yorkshire

Restricting dimensions   60' x 14'
Rise and fall   7'
Hand operated   •
Boater operated   •
Windlass required   •
Handspike required   •
Facilities nearby
⌺
Colliers Arms – 200 yards

ELLAND LOCK

Elland,
West Yorkshire

Restricting dimensions   61' x 14'
Rise and fall   7'6"
Hand operated   •
Boater operated   •
Windlass required   •
Handspike required   •
Facilities nearby

⌺ Colliers Arms – 200 yards
S Small general store
↰ 40 yards

WOODSIDE MILLS LOCK

Elland,
West Yorkshire

Restricting dimensions   60' x 14'
Rise and fall   6'6"
Hand operated   •
Boater operated   •
Windlass required   •
Facilities nearby None

LONG LEE LOCK

Salterhebble,
Halifax,
West Yorkshire

Restricting dimensions   61' x 14'6"
Rise and fall   8'
Hand operated   •
Boater operated   •
Windlass required   •
Facilities nearby None

SALTERHEBBLE LOCKS

As above

Restricting dimensions   All three locks are the
same. 60'6" x 14'
Rise and fall   Bottom 6'. Middle 9'. Top 10'
Hand operated   •
Boater operated   •
Windlass required   •
Handspike required   •
Facilities nearby
⚓
⌺ Calder & Hebble Inn – 100 yards
   Lock Head

Remarks
Open 0700 to 1800 hours.

LOCK NO. 1

Cooper Bridge,
Bradley,
Huddersfield,
West Yorkshire

Restricting dimensions   60' x 14'
Rise and fall   6'
Hand operated   •
Boater operated   •
Windlass required   •
Facilities nearby
🛢   Oil, petrol – 100 yards
⌺
Commercial – 100 yards, Three Nuns Restaurant – ¾ mile
General store, newsagent, butcher – 200 yards
↰

LOCK NO. 2

Colne Bridge,
Bradley,
Huddersfield,
West Yorkshire

Restricting dimensions   60'6" x 14'
Rise and fall   7'
Hand operated   •
Boater operated   •
Windlass required   •
Facilities nearby None

LOCK NO. 3

Bradley,
Huddersfield,
West Yorkshire

Restricting dimensions 60' x 14'
Rise and fall 5' approx.
Hand operated •
Boater operated •
Windlass required •
Facilities nearby None

LOCK NO. 4

Deighton,
Huddersfield,
West Yorkshire

Restricting dimensions 60' x 14'
Rise and fall 5'6"
Hand operated •
Boater operated •
Windlass required •
Facilities nearby None

LOCK NO. 5

As above

Restricting dimensions 59' x 14'
Rise and fall 5' approx.
Hand operated •
Boater operated •
Windlass required •
Facilities nearby None

LOCK NO. 6

As above

Restricting dimensions 59' x 14'
Rise and fall 6'6"
Hand operated •
Boater operated •
Windlass required •
Facilities nearby None

LOCK NO. 7

As above

Restricting dimensions 57' x 14'
Rise and fall 5'6"
Hand operated •
Boater operated •
Windlass required •
Facilities nearby None

LOCK NO. 8

As above

Restricting dimensions 59' x 14'
Rise and fall 6'6"
Hand operated •
Boater operated •
Windlass required •
Facilities nearby None

LOCK NO. 9 (RED DOLES LOCK)

Red Doles Lane,
Deighton,
Huddersfield,
West Yorkshire

Restricting dimensions 60' x 14'
Rise and fall 5'
Hand operated •
Boater operated •
Windlass required •
Facilities nearby

🛢 Oil, petrol – ½ mile to main road
☎ 800 yards

Details of distances and restricting dimensions are given above, and those readers who have an appropriate craft and wish to pursue an interest in this final arm are recommended to read the *Guide to the Calder & Hebble Navigation* and the *Huddersfield Broad Canal*, published by the Calder Navigation Society.

The Selby Canal

Now we do begin to enter the world of backwaters: although this stretch of waterway cannot begin to compete with probably the best known of them all, the Walton Backwaters in Essex (made even more famous by Arthur Ransome in *Secret Water*), nevertheless it should not be underestimated for it does possess some of the most secluded and attractive locations in the whole of the northeast waterways. And thereby hangs a tale, and ay, there is the rub: ever since the last commercial traffic used the canal, it has been slowly becoming more and more difficult to navigate due to the classic problems of silt and weed. Once upon a time, the dimensions for the River Aire & Selby Canal were 78' x 17'6" x 8' (air draught) with no mention of water depth; then again they

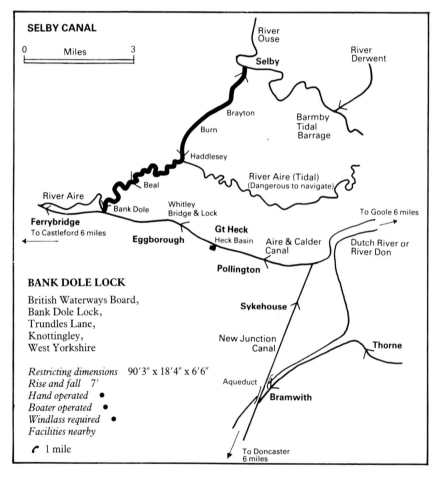

SELBY CANAL

0 Miles 3

River Ouse

River Derwent

Selby

Brayton

Burn

Barmby Tidal Barrage

Haddlesey

River Aire (Tidal)
(Dangerous to navigate)

Beal

River Aire

Bank Dole

Whitley Bridge & Lock

To Goole 6 miles

Ferrybridge
To Castleford 6 miles

Eggborough

Gt Heck
Heck Basin

Aire & Calder Canal

Dutch River or River Don

Pollington

BANK DOLE LOCK

British Waterways Board,
Bank Dole Lock,
Trundles Lane,
Knottingley,
West Yorkshire

Sykehouse

New Junction Canal

Thorne

Restricting dimensions 90'3" x 18'4" x 6'6"
Rise and fall 7'
Hand operated •
Boater operated •
Windlass required •
Facilities nearby

Aqueduct

Bramwith

⌒ 1 mile

To Doncaster 6 miles

were 78'6" x 16'6" x 6' (water) x 10' (air). The actual situation seems to be that headroom (at 12' beam) is restricted to 7' and that water draught should not really exceed 3', unless you want to risk a thoroughly hairy time. With regard to length, 78' is still theoretically O.K., but you will have serious problems of manoeuvring if you are much more than 35' at best since the possibilities of turning are severely restricted.

The best plan, if you are considering the short cut that gets you from Knottingley to Selby without having the slog of the 'outside' leg up the Ouse and the negotiation of the locks and tides at each end, is to confer with the lock-keepers at Selby and Bank Dole (Louis and Helen respectively, both persons of great worth and character). They will advise you of what is what at the time; and that is what matters since this particular canal is little used and can deteriorate from week to week.

If ever there was a candidate for betterment, or a suitable case for treatment, it must be the Selby Canal. It is not in too bad a state at the time being, and if plans were put into operation right now, it would soon become a splendid resort for those who want to get afloat and away and hide in the middle of some of Yorkshire's quietest countryside replete with bird and other wildlife. Nowhere on the waterway are you far away from anything, but, by the same token, nowhere are you very near to anything either. If you want the busy world, there is Knottingley at one end; and if you want more refined delights, Selby is at the other. Personally I find them equally attractive and have spent many happy days in both; but if I had to vote I would give the prize to Selby mainly for its market and generally better shopping facilities.

Final word of warning: if you do draw more than 3', do check with the lock-keepers about what traffic has been through recently. I have been told by a number of 'experimental' skippers that they have got through Selby canal with boats that draw up to 5'6"; only to find that when I have asked the lock-keepers if they have penned through such-and-such a boat, they have no record or recollection of it.

The entrance from Knottingley is straightforward and you will be locked on to make connection with the River Aire again. The navigation then takes a meandering course by Willow Garths, Kellingley Crook and Wood Holmes before it arrives at the weir, lock and small village of Beal where there are minimal facilities, one of which, however, is a pub. The weir comes after the bridge when you are on passage from Knottingley and boats then keep to the right for the lock. Then comes more fascinating names: Adam's Nook, Humble Holme and all the Haddleseys – West, Chapel and East – together with all the Ings that accompany them. The Selby Canal itself turns off to the left after West Haddlesey, for which there is no proper access from the water, while the river continues its way to the bridge, Dam and Lock Farm at Chapel Haddlesey. Most of the bridges are worth contemplating and some are worth capturing on film. The one that usually causes more aggro than pleasure is the last one before Selby: the swingbridge on the road just before the canal basin. It is kept locked by padlock and the key is with the keeper, whose office and house face one another across the lock gates by the Yorkshire Ouse. If you have not arranged a rendezvous with Louis (which you can easily do by telephone or VHF radio) you will need to tie up outside the canal approach to the basin and take the short walk to his office.

The basin is a popular place in season, but if you have any choice in the matter, it is better to get a berth towards the river end and so avoid some of the noisome hustle and bustle that can emanate from the bus 'station' near the bridge.

BEAL LOCK

Beal,
Selby,
North Yorkshire

Restricting dimensions 90'6" x 17'6" x 6'6"
Rise and fall 8'
Hand operated •
Boater operated •
Windlass required •
Facilities nearby
⚓⚓

🍺 Kings Head – 400 yards
S General store – 400 yards
✉ 400 yards
📞 400 yards

Remarks
Moorings in river but care should be taken in times of flood.

WEST HADDLESEY LOCK

West Haddlesey,
Selby,
North Yorkshire

Restricting dimensions 96'6" x 18' x 7'
Rise and fall Flood lock open in normal conditions
Hand operated •
Boater operated •
Windlass required •
Facilities nearby
⚓

🍺 Green Dragon – 1 mile
S General store – 1 mile

SELBY LOCK

The New Lock House,
Selby Lock,
Selby,
North Yorkshire

VHF channels 16 and 74

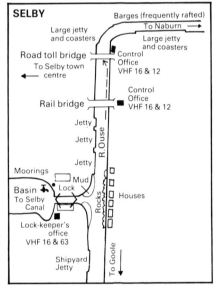

SELBY — Barges (frequently rafted)

To Naburn →

Large jetty and coasters
Large jetty and coasters

Road toll bridge
To Selby town centre ←

Control Office VHF 16 & 12

Rail bridge

Control Office VHF 16 & 12

Jetty
Jetty
Jetty

R. Ouse

Moorings
Mud
Basin ⚓
Lock
To Selby Canal

Rocks

Houses

Lock-keeper's office VHF 16 & 63

Shipyard Jetty

To Goole

Restricting dimensions 90' x 19' x 7'6"
Rise and fall Tidal
Hand operated • ⚓ 🗑 🏴
Keeper operated •   🍺 Selby town, ½ mile
Facilities nearby   S Selby town, ½ mile
                        ✉ Selby town, ½ mile
Remarks   📞 200 yards
At this tidal lock please give your estimated time of arrival to the lock-keeper (📞 Selby (0757) 703182) preferably the day before arrival.

Opening times:
Monday-Thursday 0830-1700 hours
Friday 0830-1600 hours
Saturday 0700-1200 hours
          1300-1700 hours
Sunday 0900-1200 hours
        1300-1700 hours

Short-term shelter passes for unlicensed and unregistered craft available at this location. Current details from the lock-keeper.

V. THE YORKSHIRE OUSE
The Tidal Ouse

In 1891, Tom Bradley, writing for *The Yorkshire Post*, had this to say about this Yorkshire's pride of a tideway: 'The River Ouse, that mud-stained torrent, which owns neither mouth nor source, has always played a prominent part in the country's history from the earliest times. According to Geoffrey of Monmouth, a fleet of Trojan galleys must have floated up its broad stream with the tide almost 3000 years ago, when Ebrancus, a prince of Trojan descent, is traditionally reputed to have founded the city of York by the banks of the Ouse, 980 B.C.'

In 1773, a certain Doctor Francis Drake is reported as stating: 'As early as 1080, the Conqueror's commissioners, officials and no doubt his soldiery too, travelled to and fro by the navigable waterway of the Trent and the Ouse, which was expressly called at that period the King's Way. York was very readily approached by water, the Ouse and the Trent being both tidal and in direct communication. The good men of the town of Torksey, in Lincolnshire, with their ships and other instruments of navigation, by ancient custom in lieu of paying taxes to the king, were compelled to conduct the king's officials to York. During the voyage, the High Sheriff of Yorkshire had to provide the table of the commissioners and the sailors at his own expense.'

It is true that, in one way, the mighty river does own neither mouth nor source (and, no doubt being in complete affinity with those who live near it, owes none either); but as a matter of tedious, exactitudinous fact, it actually commences at Trent Falls and ceases at a certain point when the River Ure takes over, a distance of just over 60 statute miles.

I know three rivers that share the name 'Ouse': there is the one that is the subject of this chapter; a much smaller one on the south coast that rises in Sussex and flows south into the Channel (being above Lewes hardly more than a broad stream) of 30 miles length at best; and the one that enters the Fens from The Wash a few miles below King's Lynn. This last, hardly a river deserving the description once it is entrapped in locked waters above Denver Sluice, is known as the Great Ouse, and the only reason I can offer for this epithet is one of length rather than magnitude: it is 130 miles from source to Wash, but only a short stretch of that can compete with the mighty Yorkshire Ouse and its tideway up to Naburn. To be fair, however, after much cruising of both in all kinds and conditions of river and weather, I can find little or no cause for one to seem to outshine the other whichever way your favours may lie; they are indeed both great.

Certainly the Yorkshire Ouse gets off to an impressive start, for its confluence with the Humber and the Trent, marked by the concentration camp-like tower of the Apex light, is an acreage of muddy turbulence that will impress

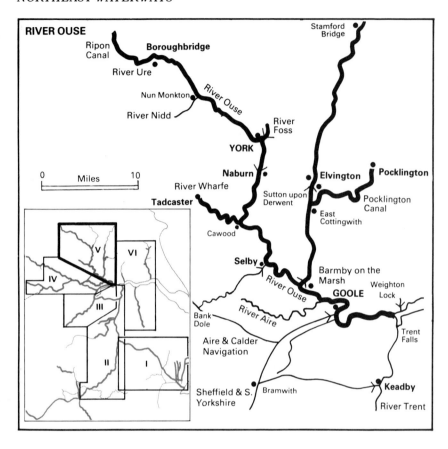

any but the most indifferent, inured or apathetic skipper and crew. It goes almost without saying that there is nothing at all apathetic about the Ouse Seaway, as the stretch from the Apex to Goole is known. To start with, Trent Falls is a bleak place at the best of times and the last time I was there was probably one of the worst of times, with a Force 9 blowing and *Valcon* without masts so as to negotiate the inland waterways, and consequently about as capable as a suet pudding of coping gracefully or even comfortably with those conditions of a northeast wind against a good spring tide. There is very little protection to be found at the confluence although there are decent anchorages in both the Trent and the Humber (see Trent Falls chart p.67) and not much more along the Seaway or the river past Goole until you have gone well on your way beyond Boothferry bridge. This knowledge should make it doubly important that anyone who thinks of cruising the lower reaches of the Ouse, and that really means downstream of Selby, should be fully equipped with a vessel that is in itself and in its equipment and crew, fully prepared for sea-going conditions.

RIVER (YORKSHIRE) OUSE

Distances
Trent Falls to Aldwark/Linton 60 miles
Trent Falls to Naburn Locks 27 miles
Naburn Locks to Aldwark/Linton 33 miles
  (non-tidal)

Dimensions
Tidal
  Length unlimited
  Beam unlimited
  Draught 6'-18' (see text)
  Air draught unlimited (bridges swing)
Non-tidal (to York)
  Length 150'
  Beam 25'
  Draught 8'
  Air draught 20'
Non-tidal (above York)
  Length 60'
  Beam 15'
  Draught 6' (see text)
  Air draught 16' (see text)

Locks 2

Traffic
There is substantial, heavy commercial coastal traffic to Goole with less to Selby and only a little heavy barge traffic to York. The rest of the waterway is used by pleasure craft of various shapes, sizes, classes and expense.

Remarks
As with the Trent, there is a vast difference between the tidal and the non-tidal reaches. Up to a mile above Selby it is essential to treat the river with the greatest of respect and only to cruise it with the same kind of craft and skills that would be applied to coastal waters. All swing bridges except Cawood can be contacted on VHF Channel 16 and use Channel 9 for working.

OS Maps (1:50 000)
105 York
  99 Northallerton and Ripon
100 Malton and Pickering

Navigation authority
Associated British Ports (Hull),
Kingston House Tower,
Bond Street,
Hull HU1 3ER
☎ (0482) 701787

(From Trent Falls to a point 100 yards below the Hook Railway Bridge.)

The Ouse Navigation Trustees,
7 St. Leonard's Place,
York YO1 2EU
Captain Rimmer, Naburn Locks
☎ (090487) 229 or 258

(From the above to 2 miles below Linton Lock).

Linton Lock Commissioners
1/3 Wheelgate,
Malton, Yorkshire.

(From the above to source.)

British Waterways Board,
Castleford Area,
Lock Lane,
Castleford, WF10 2LH
☎ (0977) 554351/5
(For the River Ure, the Ripon Canal and the Pocklington Canal)

Water authority
Yorkshire Water,
21 Park Square South,
Leeds LS1 2QG
☎ (0532) 440191

(For River Derwent)

MAXIMUM SIZES OF VESSELS

Length

Trent Falls to the tail of Naburn	Not limited
Tail of Naburn locks to York	133'
York to Swale Nab	62'

Width

Trent Falls to the tail of Naburn	Not limited
Tail of Naburn locks to York	25'
York to Swale Nab	16'

Draught

Trent Falls to Goole	
Spring tides	16'
Neap tides	9'
Goole to Selby	
Spring tides	12' (approx)
Neap tides	8' (approx)
Selby to Naburn Lock	
Spring tides	8' (approx)
Neap tides	5' (approx)
Naburn Lock to to York	9'
York to Nun Monkton Pool	6' (approx)
Nun Monkton Poole to	
Swale Nab	3'6" (approx)

Headroom beneath power cables at MHWS
Trent Falls to BOCM wharf,
Selby   75'
BOCM wharf, Selby to
Naburn Lock   60'

Headroom beneath power cables at normal
summer water level
Naburn Lock to Naburn
railway bridge   50'

Headroom beneath fixed bridge at MHWS
M62 motorway bridge   75'

Headroom beneath swing bridges at MHWS
Hook railway bridge   15'
Boothferry bridge   14'
Selby railway bridge   8'4"
Selby toll bridge :   8'9"
Cawood bridge   11'

Headroom beneath fixed bridges at normal
summer water level
Naburn railway bridge   25'
A64 (T) by-pass bridge   25'
Skeldergate bridge   23'4"
Ouse bridge   21'5"
Lendal bridge   24'4"
Scarborough railway bridge   19'5"
Clifton bridge   24'
Skelton railway bridges   24'7"
Aldwark toll Bridge   23'3"

TABLE OF DISTANCES

	Trent Falls	Blacktoft Jetty	Goole	Barmby Flood Barrier	Selby	Naburn	York	Nether Poppleton	Nun Monkton Pool	Linton	Swale Nab	Boroughbridge	Ripon	East Cottingwith	Stamford Bridge	Pocklington
Trent Falls		1	8	17	24	37	42	46	50	53	60	63	70	27	37	37
Blacktoft Jetty	1		7	16	23	36	41	45	49	52	59	62	69	26	36	36
Goole	8	7		9	16	29	34	38	42	45	52	55	62	19	29	29
Barmby Flood Barrier	17	16	9		7	20	25	29	33	36	43	46	53	10	20	20
Selby	24	23	16	7		13	18	22	26	29	36	39	46	17	27	27
Naburn	37	36	29	20	13		5	9	13	16	23	26	33	30	40	40
York	42	41	34	25	18	5		4	8	11	18	21	28	35	45	45
Nether Poppleton	46	45	38	29	22	9	4		4	7	14	17	24	39	49	49
Nun Monkton Pool	50	49	42	33	26	13	8	4		3	10	13	20	43	53	53
Linton	53	52	45	36	29	16	11	7	3		7	10	17	46	56	56
Swale Nab	60	59	52	43	36	23	18	14	10	7		3	10	53	63	63
Boroughbridge	63	62	55	46	39	26	21	17	13	10	3		7	56	66	66
Ripon	70	69	62	53	46	33	28	24	20	17	10	7		63	73	73
East Cottingwith	27	26	19	10	17	30	35	39	43	46	53	56	63		10	10
Stamford Bridge	37	36	29	20	27	40	45	49	53	56	63	66	73	10		20
Pocklington	37	36	29	20	27	40	45	49	53	56	63	66	73	10	20	

Once you are past Apex light, there is little of navigational significance until you cross over the river for the channel on the Blacktoft Jetty side. As with the Trent, there is very deep water close to the Apex light side, and the ABP chart shows quite clearly where to cross over, as do the markers and lights on the jetty. The jetty itself is quite an important staging post, not quite so much now as in the days of sail, but nevertheless still of interest to the cruising skipper.

BLACKTOFT JETTY

It is now more than thirty years since the new jetty was opened at Blacktoft. The first was built in 1873 to provide a stop-over point to help those vessels with a deeper than ordinary draught in their comings and goings up and down the river. Generally speaking, larger vessels waited in Hull Roads for about three hours after the tide had started to flood; and then they would be carried without problem of grounding or the tide turning before they reached Goole. At neap tides, and particularly if there were drought conditions with no fresh water in the river, many would in fact find themselves grounded in the Ouse. The difficulty was that they could not leave Hull any earlier without serious risk of grounding in the Humber at Whitton Sand. If they left Goole too early they would ground on the Ouse and if they left Goole too late they would ground at Whitton Sand.

Blacktoft Jetty is available to pleasure craft by permission of and at the discretion of Associated British Ports, Goole, and skippers will find that they are subject to the fourth levy as scheduled for visiting vessels. As laid down in the Ouse Lower Improvement Tolls and Rates this charge would be £6.20 for any period up to the maximum of one ebb tide. Arrangements can be made in advance by letter or telephone; alternatively the jetty master can be contacted at tide times at the jetty on VHF channel 14, and at other times the same channel can be used to make arrangements with the dock master at Goole. It must be said that while the position of Blacktoft Jetty is extremely convenient for pleasure craft (with the bonus of an easily accessible pub with grub to boot) it was nevertheless built for large commercial vessels and there is nothing about it that is not hugely built, tough and substantial. Since the wash from passing ships, coasters and barges can be considerable, in spite of the best efforts of their pilots and skippers who usually throttle back if they know small craft are moored there, it is essential to have substantial fastenings and decent lines on board your own boat. I spent one overnight stay there, and thanks to the lack of consideration of one passing coaster was faced with a repair job that cost me over £300 as planks were stove in and fittings wrenched from the deck to which they were attached, into oak, by 6″ screws.

Many people tend to use Blacktoft for better or worse – mainly for the betterment of their spirit which comes from imbibing at the local. Others search out the only additional highlight in this pretty deserted area, which is a public telephone kiosk; and perhaps it is a good idea to put in a heavy bout of socialising here, for there is little to make contact with except the waters of the Ouse after Blacktoft. The river banks do not permit many panoramic views, and even if they did, there is actually not a lot to see shoresides until you reach Goole.

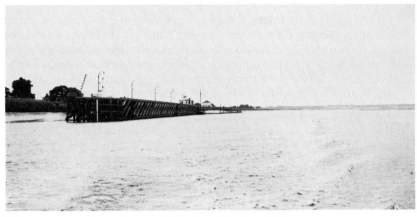

What was once a major staging post: Blacktoft and its substantial jetty.

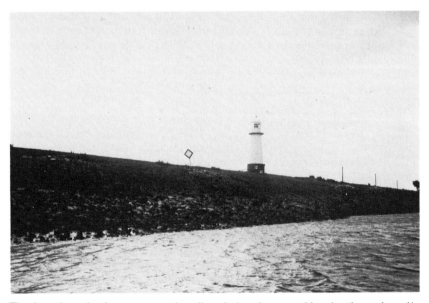

The channels on the river are extremely well marked, and any vessel keeping the marks and/or lights where they should be is unlikely to touch bottom even at low water with a draught of no more than five feet.

On the north bank there are Yokefleet and Saltmarshe; and the hall near to the latter has been the cause of much speculation about the source of the reputed millions (of pounds) in riches that someone who lived there was supposed to have amassed and scattered at least once in his lifetime. My sources have all been strong on supposition, legend and lolly, but lamentably weak on facts figures and faces. Nevertheless, it is still pleasant to muse as one passes the hall of fame.

On the south bank there are Ousefleet, Whitgift, Reedness (both Little and Large) and Swinefleet. Perhaps the most intriguingly suitable case for camera treatment is the church clock with the face that contains no XII, but instead possesses a XIII – certainly one for the book, if not for bell or candle. More importantly for the navigator however are the excellent channel markers that are clear and plain as one moves on from one ness to another; and it is good to know that, although the channels shift fairly often, the authorities at Goole have them always in their sights. The survey vessel *Ouse Patrol* is taken out from Goole docks every day to check the sounding in the bights.

While no skipper is likely to intend to navigate any of the channels at dead low water, it is nevertheless encouraging to know that, apart from exceptional conditions, a vessel drawing about three feet will be able to make safe progress while keeping strictly in the deep water channels. It is also worth noting that, in some unusual circumstances, the depth of water can be less than two feet; so it is best to work with the tides and the deeps, rather than against them.

When it comes to Goole (and when any skipper cruises up the Ouse to Ocean Lock for the first time in particular) it is abundantly manifest that it stands and falls by the docks and locks that created it, gave it life and still continue to succour it today. It is not without justice, therefore, that Associated British Ports have published a splendidly glossy brochure devoted to the promotion of the place as a major east coast port. In it, they claim the following: 'Goole is the east coast's most inland port, closer to industry than almost any other port.' Informed readers may well want to know about the claims of Selby and Gainsborough, both apparently more than 15 miles further inland than Goole, but then, perhaps, Associated British Ports have their ways of not only making mountains out of molehills but also of making statute miles out of EEC kilometres.

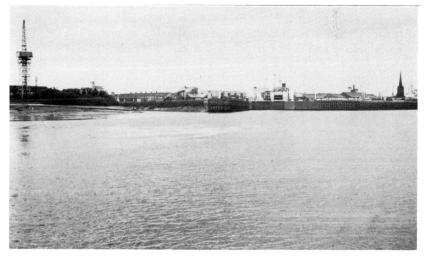

The approach to Ocean Lock, Goole, with the Dutch River to the left.

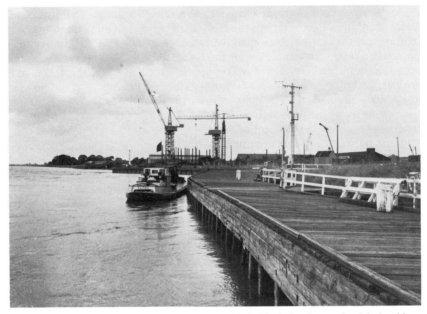

The jetty and dock signals on the riverside of Ocean Lock. The bulwarks are of such bulwarkiness that mooring and fender watches are necessary; especially when the flood or ebb may be really moving.

In any case, here we are at Goole; and whichever entrance a skipper may choose, or have chosen for him by the port operations officer of the day, he will come face to face with the awesome gates of one lock or another: Ouse, Victoria or, more probably, Ocean. The approach to all three is straightforward and uncluttered. Going upstream, Ocean Lock is the first and comes immediately after the Dutch River. This confluence with the Ouse creates quite a turbulent area of currents and cross currents, especially at the height of flow at spring tides. It doesn't make the lock inaccessible to cruising craft by any means, but it does require both skipper and craft to be sturdy and well prepared. A good ploy is to plan to arrive at the lock near the top of the tide when there will be plenty of space to manoeuvre, plenty of water to do it in, and not too much of a current to make life difficult. If you should be there when the flood or ebb are at their heights, it is important to be ready for the force that will tend to pin you against South or Middle Pier, depending upon circumstances. Further upstream, well past Middle Pier and still on the same west side of the river, come very close together the other two locks, Ouse and Victoria. For any boat's crew brought up on the locks of the Sheffield & South Yorkshire or the Aire & Calder, the locks at Goole will provide a dramatically new insight into loch control. Plenty of good sound tackle is needed and as much skill and common sense as you can muster, for while there are good men and true to assist your progress through the lock, their business is essentially to do with commercial traffic and that means big barges, tankers and ships galore. While it is true that the days are now past when many a classic 'dirty British coaster with a salt-caked smoke stack' can be spied, the spirit and the traffic remain the same.

Associated British Ports has established a Pilotage Control Centre on the Spurn Peninsula (53°44'29"N 00°06'48"E) which is constantly manned by a pilot master. This service is complemented by the 24-hour Humber Ports Operation and Information Service based at the Humber Pilot Office Building, Queen Street Hull (53°44'18"N 00°19'54"W).

Constant watch is kept on channels 16 and 12, the call sign being *VTS Humber* (Vessels Traffic Services).

The service (Tel: 0482-701787) provides information regarding the arrival, berthing, anchoring and departure of vessels and also information on navigational aids, navigation generally, visibility and the safety of vessels and persons.

Although tidal information is available, other messages will not be accepted.

In general, information on berthing, docking and other pre-arrival information is best obtained from the station serving Goole whilst navigation and safety information is obtainable from the Humber Ports Operation and Information Service.

Every two hours, commencing at 0103 hours, a general broadcast gives weather reports, tidal information and navigational warnings on channel 12, prior notification having been given on channel 16.

All vessels bound for the Humber which require the services of a Humber pilot must give 12 hours advance notice by signal through a GPO coast station to the Spurn Pilot Station (Tel: 0964 50398 Telex: 527393) giving estimated time of arrival at the seaward limits of the Humber Pilotage District and including their draught and destination.

To avoid the unnecessary interference on VHF communications encountered range, vessels wishing to communicate direct with the Spurn Pilot Station by VHF radio telephone should only call *Spurn Pilot* on VHF channel 16, and then switch to channel 14 if within about 30km.

Inward vessels wanting to pick up a Goole Pilot in Hull Roads should, giving a minimum of two hours notice of expected time of arrival, contact the Humber Ports Operation and Information Service on VHF channels 16 or 12 or through a GPO coast station or by Telex No. 527656.

Radio Information

Station	Call Sign	Channel Nos.	Operational Times	Remarks
Humber Ports Operation and Information Service, Pilot Office, 50 Queen Street, Hull	*VTS Humber*	16 12 10 13	Continuous watch maintained	Calling and safety. Navigation and safety information etc. for Rivers Humber, Ouse and Trent.
Blacktoft Jetty	*Blacktoft Jetty Radio*	16 14	3 hours before HW Goole until 1 hour after HW Goole	Calling and safety. Port Operations and berthing instructions for Blacktoft.
Goole Docks	*Goole Docks Radio*	16 14	Continuous watch maintained	Calling and safety. Port Operations and docking instructions for Goole.

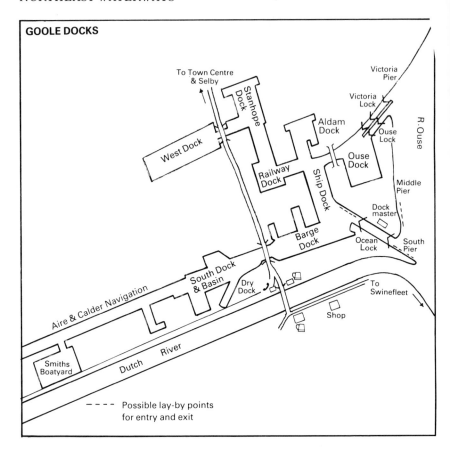

GOOLE DOCKS

GOOLE

Leeds 34 miles
Wakefield 31 miles
Sowerby Bridge 52 miles
Trent Falls 8 miles

Moorings

There are waiting moorings controlled by ABP
Goole, both inside and outside the locks; the
most usual one for yachts and pleasure craft
being Ocean Lock. ☎ Goole (0405) 2691

Marina

Smiths Boatyard: on the canal side on the way
out of Goole. The marina accepts boats of up to
6'6" draught; but for repairs can accommodate
300' x 16'6".
All facilities except petrol. ☎ Goole (0405)
3985. The principal is Mr. Heppenstall.

Boatyard

As above. But BWB also has a main office and
yard here. ☎ Goole (0405) 3631.

Club

Goole is positively jumping with clubs, but not
one is in any way connected with an ordinary
cruising club.

Facilities

🔧 ⛽ only in the town   ● ⚓ ✕ ⌂ 🚽 S
✉ ✆

Remarks

Goole Docks are extremely busy and have no
facility to entertain visiting pleasure craft.

Goole Docks Ocean Lock – Docking Signals

Day	Night		Signification
	☆ Green		
	☆ Red	A vessel is leaving Ocean	— No other vessel shall pass
	☆ Green	Lock and now entering the	into the area bounded on the
		tideway.	North by an imaginary line
	☆ Red	Ocean Lock is being made	drawn 90° from the signal
	☆ Green	available for a vessel to enter.	mast, and on the South by an
			imaginary line drawn 270°
			from Upper East Goole
	☆ Green	Ocean Lock is available	beacon.
W	E	for vessels to enter.	

Ouse and Victoria Locks Docking Signals

Red flag.	Red light.	Vessels may not enter lock.
Green flag.	Green light.	Vessels may enter lock.

Local Aids to Navigation

The Ouse and Foss Navigation Trustees administer the River Ouse from two miles below Linton Locks to a point 100 yards below Hook railway bridge (a distance of some 42½ miles) and they have published the following table.

River Ouse Navigation Marks

Starboard Name of Reach	Name or number of Beacon	Characteristic of light.	Port Name of Reach	Name or number of Beacon	Characteristic of light.
Skelton	Skelton	2FG(vert)			
Howdendyke	No. 1	2FG(vert)	Howdendyke Lee	No. 2	Fl.R1.s
Howdendyke	No. 3	Fl.G5s	Howdendyke Lee	No. 4	Fl.R1.5s
Lower Clot Hall	No. 5	Fl.G10s	Howdendyke Lee	Hook Road	Fl.R20s
			Lower Clot Hall	No. 6	Fl.R1.5s
			Boothferry	Aire	Fl.R1.5s
Upper Clot Hall	No. 7	Fl.G5s	Asselby Lee	No. 8	Fl.R1.5s
Asselby Lee	No. 9	Fl.G1.5s	Rusholme	No. 10	Fl.R1.5s
			Rusholme	Rusholme	Fl.R10s
Langrick	No. 13	Fl.G1.5s	Burr Wheel	No. 12	Fl.R5s
Hemingbrough Hope	No. 15	Fl.G1.5s	Langrick	No. 14	Fl.R1.5s
			Upper Hope	No. 16	Fl.R1.5s
			Barlow	No. 18	Fl.R1.5s
Upper Hope	No. 17	Fl.G1.5s	Barlow	Brown Cow	Fl.R1.5s
			Marrowbones	Thief Lane	Fl.R1.5s
No Man's Friend	No. 21	Fl.G1.5s	No Man's Friend	No. 20	Fl.R1.5s
Willow Tree	No. 23	Fl.G1.5s			

(All lights have 1.5M range)

The Ouse itself, and many of its settlements including the pre-eminent ones like York and Selby, go back into the mists of time, but Goole possesses no such far-reaching history; its roots are to be found no further back than the last 150 years or so. It was in the early 1820s that the first plans were put in hand to raise the site of the port by warping and there were to be an entrance harbour basin, a ship dock and a barge dock dredged to between 10 and 20 feet. There were to be two locks: one for river traffic and one for sea-going craft; but in fact the harbour basin became one huge lock.

The Lowther Hotel (originally the 'Banks') was built at this time. Some time ago, it was the headquarters of the Aire & Calder Company; and not long ago, during redecoration, some quite fantastic murals were revealed depicting Goole in the late 19th century. They are in what was the boardroom of the Aire and Calder Company. A gentle parlance (or parley if necessary) with the landlord will bring forth permission to photograph.

The port was officially opened on 20th July, 1826, and soon after many streets and buildings grew up. It is easily possible to perceive that Goole was a planned new town from the layout on the Ordnance Survey maps, since the streets all conform to someone's idea of a master plan. (No doubt for a master race of skippers, if not for a rat race to leave the ships, which, at that time, were coming in ever increasing hordes and, thanks to all the gods, were not of the sinking kind.)

In the summer of 1829, 93 foreign ships came to Goole as did 415 coastal vessels, and through to the mid 1880s trade thrived. For example, coal shipped from pit to Tom Pudding to hoist to ship was 15,913 tons in 1868 and was 201,949 tons in 1884. By contrast and comparison, and certainly to show that all is not ill with British commerce or the ABP operations, it can now be claimed that Goole has a tradition, albeit not as longstanding as some, of reliability, flexibility and efficiency; a claim backed up by the fact that the port handles, in a normal year, some 2,000 vessels and more than 1½ million tonnes (hardly different from a ton, and certainly not worth the effort of all those EEC Common Market letters!).

I remember Goole as if it were only yesterday; but a yesterday of a childhood that is in fact fifty light (if not light-hearted) years distant.

In those dear, dark days, sometimes best beyond recall, I was taken every ritual weekend from the vertical excesses of the steelworks chimneys of Appleby Frodingham at Scunthorpe to the horizontal panoramas of the bleak east coast at Ulrome; and, in order to get there, we used to drive round the inland route because my mother did not like to travel over water, that is, not over the gaps between the sleepers on the jetty that led to the old ferry from New Holland (now also a yesterday). In those days, Goole was a place of girdered bridges, coal dust, all-sorts dust and just dust. During the many times I have stayed there on *Valcon* over the past three years I have found little in those areas that has changed. Indeed, there is still so much dust lurking by and on the bridges that I am constantly amazed that they work as swiftly and efficiently as they do.

However, coal dust may be unpleasant to some, but to Goole it is its life blood; Goole established itself, well over 100 years ago, as one of the country's premier coal-handling ports, and it still ships coal, coke and smokeless fuels in large quantities direct from road, rail or barge transport. It also handles a wide variety of ores, chemicals, fertilisers, scrap, pitch, creosote, tar and animal feedstuffs; in addition, because it is close to crushing plants, a trade has grown in 'exotics', namely, palm nut kernels, shea nuts and other oil-bearing seeds. Such cargoes must be more than enough to cause the atmosphere to carry its fair share of foreign bodies, and so explain the presence of so much 'dust'. Nor is 'going foreign' uncommon to the port, for there is regular traffic with Iceland, Finland, Sweden, Spain, the Canary Islands, the Mediterranean ports, the Red Sea and South America.

However, there is nothing exotic about another equally regular import/export, and that is the effluent that is brought in tankers and bunkered into a ship and taken out to sea. No doubt there are those will say unequivocally that nothing of that kind should be dumped at sea; my view is closer to home: the effluent operation is very close to the repair depot of the British Waterways Board and, on one occasion when I was working the area, BWB were kind enough to let me moor there for a few days. I still ask myself, 'Was it a kindness', for the stench that overcame me when the wind veered slightly was quite out of this world. Those who work near to it, but not with it, refer to it as a 'whiff', but that must be misleadingly euphemistic for an odour that seems to combine the worst excesses of sugar beet factory chimneys and commercial disinfectants. Most cruising skippers will not be forced into close confrontation with any continuing pong, since most will come through one of the locks and then move to the further reaches of the Aire & Calder unless they are going to stay for a while and enjoy the marina facilities of Smith's Boatyard; a business that has been there for some long time, and which, happily, shows no sign of not continuing to do so for many years to come.

Both upstream and downstream, both course and channel bend, twist and turn (and not always in the same direction as each other); while the river bed rises and falls as much as ten metres in depth in as many feet in length, creating a plethora of boils, slacks, eddies and runs. It is a foolhardy skipper who goes out there without someone to guide his efforts at his first attempt. As long ago as 1828 the sub commissioners for pilotage at Kingston-upon-Hull agreed to examine and license pilots for the Lower Ouse; and it was resolved by the brethren that 6 pilots might operate between Hull Roads and Goole. Today, the pilots are licensed by Associated British Ports at Hull and there are 14 based there and 12 based at Goole, working the big ships up and down the river respectively.

'In a calm sea every man is a pilot'; but there are many occasions when the waters up to and around Goole are anything but calm, and anyone having watery business at that time can be confident that the pilots (whether Hull/Goole or Goole/Hull, and whether in the locks and docks or on the river) will serve and protect Goole and its traffic to the best of their canny ability. All pilots are a race apart; and there is nothing about the Goole pilots that makes them any less men of individual, incorrigible character than the rest.

When going upstream from Goole to Selby or Naburn it is important not to leave too soon; and for any craft drawing a touch more than three feet that means no earlier than one hour after the flood has reached Goole. Even then you should still take it easy once out on the river since any show of speed will only have you encountering the bottom at any number of places after Hook railway bridge. For those who have not personally experienced the power of a

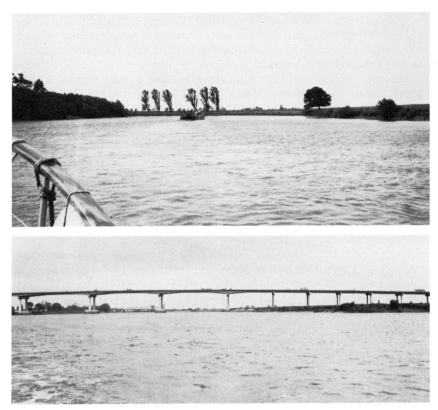

The two extremely noticeable features on the river above Goole: the six poplars that are mentioned in almost everything that has been written about the Ouse; and the 'new' road bridge (Ouse Bridge) above Boothferry.

spring flood up the stern when the bows are in the mud, let me plead with them not to try, since there is a very good chance that the craft will founder, having a deep pit scoured beneath her keel and turned into it in no time at all. I have, as a result of foolishly having given in to the demands of impatience and left too soon on the flood on the King's Lynn Ouse, been caught in such straits and now vow never to risk such possible disasters again.

The channel follows the usual disciplines, keeping to the outside of the bends and the sketch map shows in general terms what this means in the tricky area from below Hook to above Asselby. (Those readers who would like to study the matter in even more detail are referred to the *Cruising Guide* published by the Ripon Motor Boat Club.) While it is always sensible to give the nesses wide berths, it is also important on this river to keep well clear of the 'rubble-trouble' that can be expected close to the banks on the outsides of some of the turns. There can be no more than the usual hazards of rubbish that cause foul bottoms on many of our rivers; but there can be tips and dumps, irrespon-

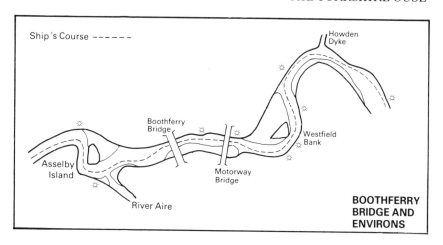

Ship's Course ------

Howden Dyke

Boothferry Bridge

Westfield Bank

Asselby Island

Motorway Bridge

River Aire

BOOTHFERRY BRIDGE AND ENVIRONS

sibly placed far too close to the riverside, that simply build up too much and then fall down the bank; and the dangerous remains of piles and stakes that once upon a time were useful but for many a long year have outlived their function and now lurk to catch out the unwary navigator.

So; the principle on this river must therefore be to tend to keep to the outside of the bends, but not to overdo it, and to try to read the waters accurately so that shoal patches are completely avoided. However, one should not rely on visual observations that clash with a definite reading from a properly operational depth sounder.

There are two dramatic aspects in this area. The first is the tremendous acreage of water that exists at Howden Dyke Island which may tempt the newcomer to take a course straight ahead instead of the marked 90 degree turn to port that is the course of the ebb channel. True, there is a 'flood' channel straight across, but it is only for those who know the river well and have a vessel that draws not much more than three feet. Just as in rounding any headland out at sea, it seems to take so long to get round, that the corner after the Tate & Lyle jetties appears to be ready to defeat you by squaring the circle and leading you astray. Strict attention to the chart and the wheel must be the order for the day.

The second attention-grabber must be the vision of the old and new bridges known respectively as Boothferry and Ouse. Indeed, the latter has achieved such fame that it now graces the cover of the Ordnance Survey Routemaster map of the East Midlands and Yorkshire (Sheet 6). They both dominate the river from a long way downstream, and offer many changing attitudes, perspectives and façades, all of which are impressive. The photography enthusiast should make sure that he is not clobbered inexorably at the wheel for this stretch.

Not far upriver from here comes the tidal barrage that marks the entrance to the River Derwent (please refer to pp.213-217) and about five miles further up comes Selby. The approach to the stretch which contains the lock and the two bridges is fairly straight; in fact, the town and the abbey can be seen from some distance away. This is more than can be said for the lock since it is set well back and will not reveal itself until you are almost past it. However, there are some unmistakable signs: Selby shipyard is on the left just below the lock, and on the opposite bank the first development of houses 'proper' are almost over-looking the lock entrance.

The resident lock-keeper, Louis, runs a tight lock and a friendly basin with no unnecessary leaks, likes or dislikes. He is to be relied on well beyond the call of duty. He can be contacted by telephone, Selby (0757) 703182, or VHF radio, channels 16 and 74. See page 176 for details.

The drill he recommends for entering the lock is to stem the tide and to make sure that he has actually seen you. The chances are that he will have done so anyway, but checking like this means categorically that you are in touch. It is best to stem the tide from a position upstream of the lock – not downstream. The reason is, that, should you get into any difficulty, if you are above the lock, level with the keeper's house – although you may not be able to see it from your craft, he will stand a decent chance of getting a rope to you; whereas, if you are downstream of the entrance, the chances are really very slim.

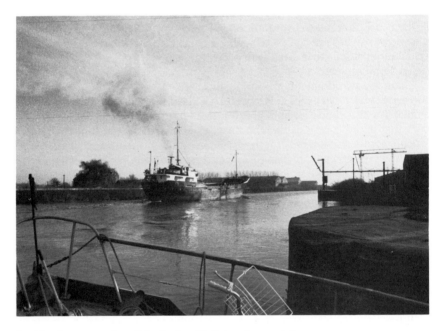

Looking downstream from Selby Lock, with *Valcon* about to follow a coaster.

Whether you are proposing to enter from above or below the lock it is important to make your last approach from a course that tends to the lock side of the river. On each side of the entrance there are soft mudbanks; but on the opposite side of the river, the banks and bottom both above and below the entrance are foul with rocks and other unpleasant items.

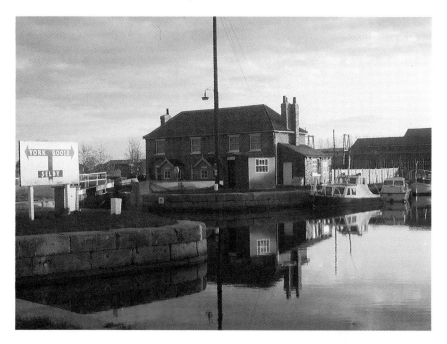

The old lock cottages are a joy to view in the basin at Selby. The 'new' house for the lock-keeper is out of the picture to the left, but his office can be clearly seen in the centre.

The bridges at Selby are also a cause for special concern, consideration and mention. Firstly, the run up to both bridges can be complicated by the presence of up to three coasters moored abreast, above and below the bridges; and the big ships at the BOCM jetties, with the many barges across the other side, can cause extreme variations in the currents, especially at anything less than high water. It is currents that cause the other major difficulty: when there is a good spring tide and/or flood water on the river, only those with the stoutest of tackle and soundest of engines should venture anywhere near the bridges, since the tows are such that there is no room for manoeuvre if in trouble, and very little even when not. (Selby bridges, or anywhere on the tidal Ouse for that matter, is no place for risking a Sunday afternoon swannee down the river in a lightweight cruiser powered by a 4HP outboard motor.)

There are bye-laws governing the negotiation of the bridges at Selby. Since they are exclusively concerned with the safe passage of all and sundry through them, they are given in full below.

Selby Toll Bridge

a. No master of a vessel exceeding 9.50 metres in extreme breadth shall pass Selby toll bridge except with the consent in writing of the Trustees.

b. Subject to the provisions of paragraph (a) of this bye-law no master of a vessel shall pass Selby toll bridge except
   (i) at slack water or against the stream or (ii) going astern with the stream

c. Notwithstanding the provisions of paragraph (b) of this bye-law no master of a vessel exceeding 50 metres in length or 8.75 metres in extreme breadth shall pass Selby toll bridge going astern with the stream except with the consent of the Trustees, which shall be obtained by the master of a vessel exceeding 9.50 metres in extreme breadth in addition to that required under paragraph (a) of this bye-law.

Calling, listening out, and contact between bridge and ship stations to be established on channel 16. Immediately thereafter transfer is to be made to the working frequency, which is channel 9, with channel 12 as an alternative.

Vessels inward bound to call Selby rail bridge 10 minutes before estimated time of arrival at that bridge; vessels outward bound to call Selby toll bridge 10 minutes before estimated time of arrival at that bridge.

Vessel to call on channel 16, giving her name and working frequency. Irrespective of which bridge is being called both bridges to reply confirming working frequency, the bridge being called to reply first.

Vessel to repeat call on working frequency and state whether inward or outward bound, and whether one or both bridges are to be opened.

Both bridges to acknowledge understanding of vessel's requirements, and all stations to remain on working frequency until vessel's manoeuvre through the bridges is complete.

If one bridge fails to answer a vessel's call the other bridge may answer in lieu, after establishing land line communication with the non-answering bridge.

The system whereby vessels request the bridges to open by means of 1 prolonged followed by 6 short blasts on the whistle or siren will continue to be used in addition to radio communication.

There is no doubt that this part of the river can be problematic; but there is also no doubt that the problems can be overcome without too much difficulty, as witness the hundreds of craft that do so every year without loss of life or limb. Nevertheless, the bridge and lockmasters are always there at tide times with an eye and an ear for possible complications. Least doubtful of all must be the charms of Selby itself; once a thriving abbey place and now something different. Once it was a centre of all kinds of religious industries (or should that be industrious religions?) and the kind of wheeling and dealing that is always associated with kings, charters and abbots.

In terms of commercial activity Selby is still doing quite well: below the toll bridge in the centre of the town, there are situated four wharves, all on the south bank. The lowest is owned by Rostron's Ltd, paper makers, but is generally not in regular use except as a lay-by berth. Just above Selby Canal there is a wharf operated by General Freight, and below the railway bridge, one run by Selby Shipping Ltd. This company also runs the newest wharf in Selby which is situated between the two bridges. Above the toll bridge (where are to be found the Ideal Flour Mills and Providence Mill) is Abbots Staith; and it is just possible that some of the original masonry from this staith still remains

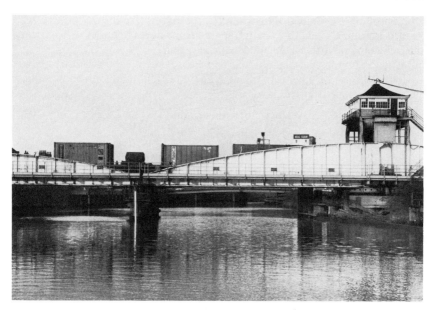

The railway bridge at Selby: a monument to *fin de siècle* style engineering.

beneath the flour mills. Upstream of Providence wharf and on the opposite bank (right 'round the bend' in fact) are the wharves of BOCM Silcock; and they are the longest continuous wharfage on the river. Up to three coasters may be handled at the same time at this wharf; but it is most often crowded with barges from Hull and from Immingham. There are also many barge moorings on the opposite side of the river from this wharfage.

This stretch must certainly rank as one of the most heavily populated and also one of the busiest on the river. At certain times it almost looks as if you could walk from one side of the river to the other without getting your feet wet so many are the craft to be found in the area. In fact, their presence can also create some quite arbitrary currents, drifts, swirls and boils, especially at low-ish water, that can be quite a threat to an unknowing skipper with a less-than-powerful small craft. However, in general the cruising man will find that skippers and crews are usually helpful, and the presence of so many barges has been for many years and for many cruising skippers a godsend when it came to finding an overnight berth that was convenient to catch the tide first thing next day. Cruising men also have cause to be grateful to the consideration of the river pilots of the commercial ships that come up the river; in general, they do all they can to cause small craft as little difficulty as possible, bearing in mind that they can manoeuvre only with difficulty and must remain in the deep water channel . . . and at a rate of knots that will give them steerage. Vessels of up to 4.8m (16 feet) get to use the lower part of Selby at spring tides and 3m (10 feet) at neap tides.

The port of Selby was also important and busy back in history: in A.D.71, Quintus Petilius Cerialis, a Roman General, came north to fight the Brigantes, and this confirmed the navigation which was already being used as a trade route, with supplies via the Witham and Fossdyke and the Trent from The Wash and through Lincoln. In about A.D.800, Alcuin, a monk and scholar, mentions the flourishing trade:

From the most distant lands ships did arrive,
And safe in port lay there, tow'd up to shore,
Where, after hardships of a toilsome voyage,
The sailor finds a safe retreat from sea.
By flow'ry meads, on each side of its banks,
The Ouse, well stoed with fish, runs through the town.

The town he mentions may well be York, but the same waters flowed through Selby, and there is no doubt that the same tides brought up the stone for the building of the abbey. This quite amazing Norman example of abbey churches that survived the dissolution of the monasteries dominates the main street and has an original 14th century window that has more impact than all the double glazing in the rest of the town. At the time of the 11th and 12th centuries the abbey was rich beyond the dreams of abbesses with many possessions in the marshland villages at Whitgift and Reedness. Apart from these monastic doings, to-ings and fro-ings, the main trade through Selby was in cloth and shipbuilding.

In 1698 Selby had been known as the 'place upon ye Ouze to which most goods either imported from abroade or to be exported thither are now brought.' The Selby Canal was opened in 1778 and any decline in trade was halted, and in 1800 800 coasters a year were coming through. There was also an upsurge in passenger traffic: the *Joanna* left Selby for Hull and all stations on the Ouse and Humber every Monday morning, returning on Thursdays. The fare was 2/- single and meals were 6d for 'men', but only 4d for 'women'.

In 1791 the Selby Bridge Act was passed, laying down maximum tolls and declaring that vessels should always have the right of way. The toll bridge is still carrying on the tradition even to this day. In 1840 a railway bridge made in cast iron was opened but it was too narrow and dangerous on big tides. It was replaced in 1891 by the present swing bridge. Even today, things have changed very little here, since the bridges still are a cause for concern and special consideration whether you approach by land or water.

The well-kept and attractive basin is quite close to the town and very close to grocery and hostelry, although the 'short cut' by the lock-keeper's house is an alley way that goes through territory that is often littered with refuse and muddily difficult to negotiate. Nearby, however, there is a touch of olde-worlde: the old cottages by the lock add an air of heritage and nostalgia; and for those who want to venture into town, I would recommend three matters that are well worth an extra day's stay-over if necessary: market day, with a gathering that spreads apparently far and wide through the town and into all kinds of nooks and crannies; the wet fish shop in the square opposite the post office, where you will find fish not only to your taste, but also to your pocket; and the Selby Bookshop, by the traffic lights at the 'other' end of town, where they will not only sell you books, but will also refrain from doing so if that is what seems seemly . . . and will also offer you advice, help, comment and conversation. In fact, all that a good bookshop should do; long may they continue in their fair trading, which has nothing at all to do with wheeling and dealing.

Timing when to leave Selby Lock, to go up or downstream will depend very much upon your power, your draught and your skills. The flood of a spring tide can shift the water through the bridges at anything up to 8 knots, so many skippers will want to wait until just before high water, when the main force will be spent. This timing will mean not only a calm passage through the arches but also plenty of water under the keel all the way to Naburn which is nearly fifteen miles distant. However unless you know the river and its circumstances well, the best plan is to let the lock-keeper know the details of your craft, together with a realistic assessment of your ability, and ask for his advice about how and when to leave. In addition, he will be able to 'read' the fresh flood water conditions if they exist at that time and vary his advice accordingly. Similar timings apply if you intend to head down the river for the Derwent through Barmby tidal barrage, a distance of about six miles.

Passing the tollbridge on your way upstream, you may well find yourself being courteously waved along your way by one or more of the staff. They are all of a breed that could fill a list of characters from a *fin de siècle* chronicle of the everyday stories of bridge folk; while they reign at the bridge there will be little threat to its unique character or heritage.

After this bridge comes the vast bend where, when the tides really run, powerful 'boils' indicate the state of the turbulence followed by the BOCM jetties and the barge parks. The stretch is straight and straightforward except for the slight oddities in current speeds and directions that can be caused by the arrangements of so many tied up vessels and leads finally to the last bend out of Selby with a 90 degree turn to port into Barlby Reach, and it is from this point that the river takes on an entirely new visage. Downstream of Selby, the Ouse is marked mainly as a wide and muddy waterway with little to relieve the visual monotony of wide and muddy banks. After Barlby though, the scenery becomes, if neither truly rural nor a riparian's delight, then at least more decorative and attractive than it has been before. It continues in this manner until Naburn, and since there is little to threaten or challenge on this leg except the on going encounters with all kinds, shapes and sizes of floating hazards coming downstream in bits and pieces or in nasty 'islands' or hordes everyone on board will have a good chance to pass by and stare.

After Turnhead farm, there is no safe mooring until Naburn except for the pontoons at Cawood belonging to the water-ski club, which are, by repute, most zealously and jealously guarded by the membership and from which you should expect to be moved on. There is a bridge that swings at Cawood normally with 11' for air at mean high water springs but if you are in any doubt,

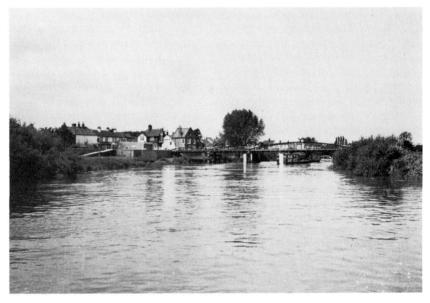

Cawood: the bridge with its arches clearly marked up for navigation.

you should ring the keeper before you set off and try to agree a strategy if not an actual timing. Legend has it that he responds to the ship's whistle. Legend also informs that the huge bridge at Kingsferry on the River Swale in Kent will respond to a bucket in the rigging but it doesn't. A prior telephone call, Cawood (075 786 217) is altogether more reliable. The village presents a most appealing aspect to the river and it is sad that there is no facility for landing at any stage of the tide.

Just above Cawood is one of Yorkshire's pride and joys: the River Wharfe of Wharfedale fame. There is a noticeable 'pull' as you pass Wharfe's Mouth (no less symbolic than real) and cruisers that draw no more than a metre should be able to navigate up to Tadcaster on a good spring tide. I delicately pushed *Valcon's* nose into the mouth once, and found that, even on top of the tide, there was so little room for manoeuvre with her draught that it would have been folly to have ventured further in spite of the recommendations for the local brew at the head of the navigation. The river is said to take its name from the Saxon, *guerf*, meaning 'swift', and there is little doubt that it can be that, as shown by the great floods of 1686 which carried away most of the bridges and buildings right down the valley. It drains a good deal of Yorkshire, starting on Cam Fell in Langstrothdale and using up nearly seventy miles to get to its junction with the Ouse.

There is now only one place before Naburn to catch the eye, and that is the small community of Acaster Selby. Once upon a time, it was the headquarters of all kinds of commerce and traffic, but now all it offers to the boater's eye is a rare collection of geese – certainly not to be despised however. At this stage in the cruise though, it will be the approach, weir and locks at Naburn that will figure most in the mind. There is a straight stretch, much favoured by fishermen, just before the locks. The weir can be seen straight ahead and the locks are to the right. There is a spit coming out from the east bank just below the lock so it is a good plan to open up the gates fully before beginning a turn. The keepers will inform you which of the two chambers you should use. (Please see chartlets p 200 and 205).

At the time of writing, negotiations are still taking place between the Ouse & Foss Trustees and the British Waterways Board about a possible take-over. In 1985 the charge for a one-way penning was £8.00. The trustees publish bye-laws relating to the navigation of the Ouse and the Foss and the following are relevant to Naburn and other locks. It is to be noted that Naburn is the headquarters of Captain Rimmer, the river manager for the Trustees.

Mooring

Any vessel which in case of emergency has to moor temporarily in Naburn Cut shall not moor alongside any dredger or hopper or any other vessel belonging to the trustees.

Every vessel at anchor below Naburn Locks shall have its anchor buoyed.

No person shall cut any mooring line or unmoor or cut adrift any vessel.

Except in an emergency no person shall moor or fasten a vessel to any fence, tree, bridge, lock, drain, dam, weir, clough or any other works not specifically provided for mooring or fastening vessels.

Locks

No vessel shall be penned through any lock owned or operated by the Trustees except by or with the consent of an authorised officer of the Trustees.

The master of a vessel shall not enter or attempt to enter leave or remain in a lock except with the consent of an authorised officer of the Trustees and in accordance with the conditions of such consent.

No person shall

a. Use any fender shod with iron or other metal against the lock gates or other works in the navigation.

b. Interfere with any lock gate, lock clough, sluice, bywash or dam.

c. Moor a vessel in or within 45 metres of any lock or bridgeway without the consent of the Trustees.

d. Place a vessel so as to obstruct the passage of any other vessel into or out of any lock or enter any lock out of turn.

e. Suffer a vessel to remain at the mouth of any basin, bridgeway, lock, drain, cut or dock longer than is necessary by passing.

f. Navigate a vessel into or out of a lock before the relevant lock gates are open to their full extent.

The locks at Naburn, like their guardians and operators, are real gems; there is nothing about them that indicates a passion for the contemporary, the avant garde, the automated or the remote controlled. Everything here goes at a proper human pace and with a real regard for the true nature of boats, boaters and water. However, in the interests of fair play and decent treatment all round, let me also add that it will not be a waste of time to make sure that your craft is well dressed overall with stout fenders (though not so stout that they will offend the bye-laws that prohibit the use of ferrous metals for such purposes!). There is no immediate riverside community or facility at the locks so a short trip upstream is required before you can achieve the luxury of a bankside mooring outside a pub. If you are lucky, you will be passed through

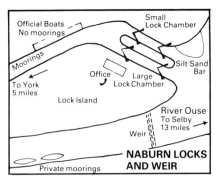

NABURN LOCKS
AND WEIR

Facilities
Acaster ⚓ 🛢 ● ✕ ⌷ ♩S ⚓

Naburn ⚓ 🛢 ● ⚓ ♩S ⛽

Remarks
Cawood to Naburn. Shallow in patches – catching tide essential.

NABURN

Moorings
Naburn Marina Ltd has a considerable number for hire.

Marinas
Naburn Marina Ltd – east side of river
Naburn, York YO1 4RW
☎ (0904) 21021
Acaster Marine Ltd – west side
Intake Lane, Acaster Malbis, YO2 1UL
☎ Escrick (0904) 706819

Boatyard
Naburn Marina Ltd.

Club York Motor Boat Club

NABURN LOCKS

☎ Escrick (0904) 87229 and (0904) 87258

Restricting dimensions Large. 133' x 24'6"
Small 82'6" x 19'6"
Rise and fall Large 9'. Small 9'
Hand operated ●
Keeper operated ●
Boater operated ●
Facilities nearby
⚓
⌷ 1 mile
✉ 1 mile (opening limited)
Remarks
Small lock opened 1756. Large lock opened 1888.
Castle Mills Lock, River Foss, York 97' x 18'6" x 6'6" x 10'

the locks by Captain Rimmer himself, as spick-and-span as if on the bridge of the *Queen Mary* and with that brand of politesse that goes with it. The experience will be a right and proper introduction to the rich, the riches and the richness that are to be found upstream of the locks, which is, in very truth, a land symbolically flowing with milk and honey. It will take no more than a glance at the sides of the river, which are around here things of sculpted, landscaped splendour with nary a blade of grass out of its lacquered place, to convince you that you are entering a promised land, but promised by whom to whom being a well kept secret. Should you gaze for long on the monuments to what real money can do when invested in a riverside property, you will immediately begin to understand why it is important to cruise this stretch with respect for its *genius loci*, which in this case combines a sense of place with a deference to filthy lucre.

The first village community comes on the port hand, on the west bank, and is Acaster Malbis. It is quaint in many ways, but particularly in possessing a quite landlocked boatyard/marina with access along a country lane. There is a pontoon for the clientele of the Ship, but it is only a satisfactory berth if your draught is no more than 1.5m. There is also a small slipway nearby. On the

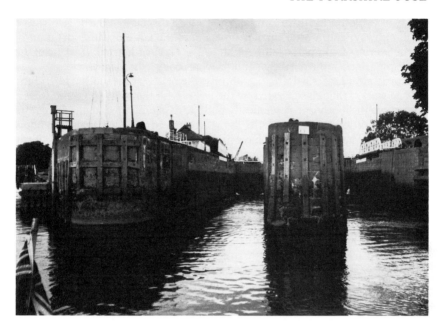

The two locks at Naburn: large one to the left; smaller one to the right.

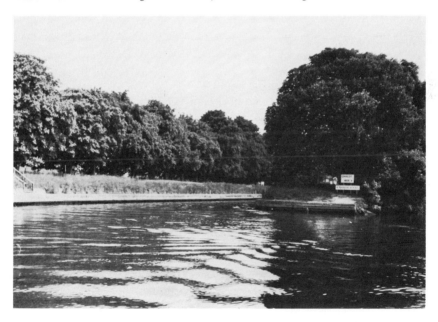

Above the lock at Naburn, looking back with the lock to the left and the weir to the right.

opposite bank not far upstream lies the actual village of Naburn, also with a small slipway, and a little further up again is the large marina operation of Yacht Services Ltd., perhaps better known as Naburn Marina. It is one of the biggest marinas in the northeast and provides comprehensive services.

Shortly after comes a dramatic contrast: the palace at Bishopthorpe and the sewage works; though separated by the river, with the palace going to west if not waste. Bishopthorpe is scenically poised, rising, on a bend and in a quite superior position; with the works discreetly placed as a sign that they know their place. The lords spiritual have in this instance got the better of the lords temporal and they can look down on the scene below, quoting Ozymandias the while: 'Look on my works, ye Mighty, and despair!' and no doubt in his time every bishop has contemplated the nature of that infinite wisdom that saw fit to place his station just above the works of the world, the flesh and the devil; and those readers familiar with John Whiting's play, *The Devils*, will know just how much poetically licensed mileage he was able to get out of the confluence of high church and low sewer. Whatever your stance may be, it is difficult not to see the place as a setting ideally suited to grand matters of state and estates and just crying out for the Coming (be it first or second) of the Good, the Great, the High and the Mighty by punt, launch or barge.

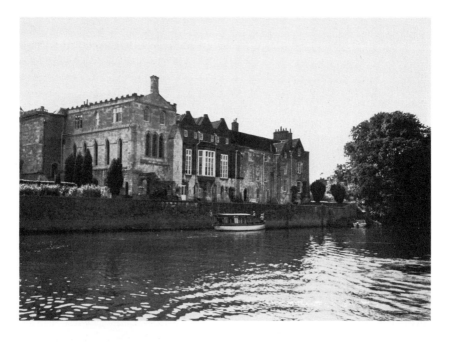

The Palace at Bishopthorpe; where the incumbent is by no means recumbent in posture – be it physical or metaphysical. However, he is fairly well protected from waterborne marauders since there is little depth by this patch.

By this time, the York bypass, the A64, is ready to heave into view marking the onset of Fulford and the headquarters of the hospitable York Motor Yacht Club, with, close by, the outposts of the athletically inclined rowing clubs, whose members seem not to be aware of the meaning of any sound signals, or if they are, tend to treat them as if they have no meaning, for they can shout as bold as brass at any whistle, dismissing it as if it were no more than the echo of a tinkling cymbal. Indeed, not even the charitable tongues of men and angels can deter them from the rigid attitudes and courses that their obsessive competitive postures force them to adopt.

The first signs of York proper come with the bridges and the unmistakable chimney of the glass factory that stands, as if a sentinel, by the River Foss and its controlling lock, Castle Mills. Passage through this lock can be achieved, after some considerable parley and negotiation, part of which is a cripplingly high penning fee, with Captain Rimmer, the river manager, and for those who are not content until they have floated through every single inch of any remotely navigable waterway, there is no doubt the great attraction of the short stretch that gives access to part of York's soft and remarkably attractive underbelly. Most boating folk will, quite understandably, be content to creep into the basin, turn round and come out again; sussing out York's beauty spots by foot and not by Foss.

The bridges are a great attraction also, and not only to those who come to cruise under them or to walk or drive over them, or even to peer over their stonework, but also to those with predilections for hanging from niches, shouting from lamp posts, and jumping from edges – with or without having previously displayed the naked cheeks of their nether regions to whomsoever they may be of concern. Many admiring or despairing but either way attentive glances focus on them and this encourages them and their camp followers. I have found that a reasonably good way to avoid suffering their outrages is to avoid the bridges at weekends; and if you are really keen to miss out on them, then to cruise the area only in the winter. The fortnight I once spent in midwinter moored at King's Staithe was an absolutely idyllic time, when my only regular contact with life (human or otherwise) was a morning visit from a lame duck for his warm bread and milk breakfast; visiting the same spot at the height of the summer season was a surprise and a real disappointment. I prefer the memories of frosty mornings with palely lit bridges.

There are five big bridges spanning the Ouse at York. Going upstream, they are: Skeldergate, Ouse, Lendal, Scarborough and Clifton. Probably the first bridge in York was the Roman one on the site of the present Ouse bridge. It was discovered in 1893 and was originally made of wood on stone piers. There was also a mediaeval bridge, first mentioned just after the Norman Conquest, and this 13th century bridge was of stone with shops and houses built on it. The present bridge was opened in 1830. The present Lendal bridge was opened in 1863, Skeldergate in 1881 and the single-span road bridge at Clifton in 1963.

Since volume after volume could be written about the city of York (be it of today, yesterday or tomorrow) there is little point in trying here to say anything

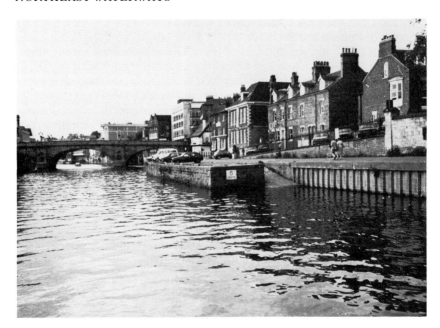

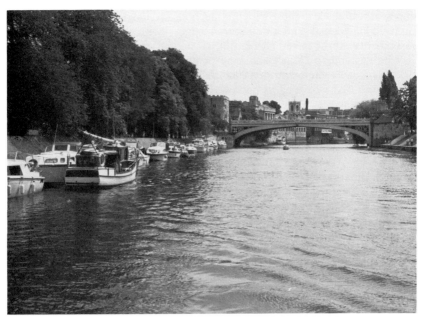

Views and popular mooring possibilities in the centre of York.

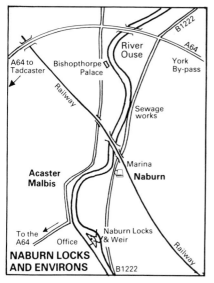

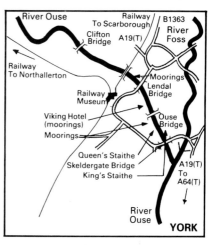

YORK

Moorings
There are public moorings (by grace and favour of the council) in York; and visitors are welcome as below.

Marina
Yacht Services Ltd , Naburn. Naburn Marina.

Boatyard
Acaster Marine, Naburn Marina and Hill's Cruisers can be called on to help in an emergency in York.

Club
York Motor Yacht Club, Fulford (just downstream of York itself).

Facilities
(If not actually within the city walls then very close by.)

Remarks
The only real hazards are to be your time and your pocket; both of which are likely to be severely raided but to excellent purpose. York has everything needed for leisure and pleasure, though strictly boating-orientated services are not a speciality.

other than it is a fantastic place for a stop over – for an hour or two, or a year or two; there are all the amenities and facilities that any cruising family could ask for, with specialist boat needs attended to just down the river at the boatyards. There are also bye-laws as promulgated by the trustees of the Ouse and Foss Navigation, and an extract from these is given below.

A vessel at anchor or lying at any quay, wharf, staith, pier, jetty, landing, mooring or river bank shall at all times be kept properly and effectually secured and made fast.
The master of any vessel which is berthed at a quay, wharf, staith, pier, jetty, landing, mooring or river bank shall ensure where necessary that satisfactory means are provided for safe access to and from the vessel.

a. Except in case of emergency no vessel shall moor or remain moored alongside any quay, wharf, staith, pier, jetty, landing or river bank without the permission of the person for the time being in charge of such quay, wharf, staith, pier, jetty, landing or river bank.

b. A vessel not loading or discharging a cargo shall not be left moored or anchored in any

205

part of the river other than at a private wharf or private landing except with the consent of the Trustees, provided that and without prejudice to the provisions of paragraph (c) of this bye-law the consent of the Trustees need not be obtained to moor at any public mooring or landing.

c. No pleasure boat shall remain at any public mooring or landing for a period exceeding 48 hours without the consent of the Trustees.

d. No pleasure boat shall moor at public moorings or landings within the City of York for longer than 48 hours in any period of seven days (beginning with the time at which the pleasure boat first moored at any such mooring or landing within the city) without the consent of the Trustees. Periods of waiting by a pleasure boat at more than one public mooring or landing within the city shall be aggregated together for the purposes of this paragraph.

A person using a vessel, on arriving at a mooring place, shall moor the vessel in such a position and in such a manner as (a) to prevent any risk of injury to any other vessel or its mooring and (b) to cause no obstruction to the safe convenient access to another vessel, or to the safe and convenient embarkation or disembarkation therefrom.

A vesssel left moored or anchored at any public wharf, staith, river walk, pier, jetty, landing or mooring with or without the consent of the Trustees and left unmanned must have displayed in a conspicuous position the master's name and address and if available telephone number at which he may be contacted.

The city council allows free mooring along this stretch of river for up to 48 hours at a time. The council also provides a free water point and waste disposal point (both sewage and refuse) for river users adjoining the public toilets at Lendal Bridge as shown below:

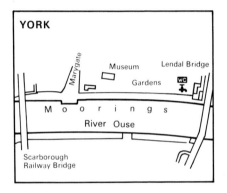

Should you want to escape from the delights of York, you can do so quite easily upriver where in no time at all you will be away from it all, past the National Railway Museum, past the sugar beet factory and on to Clifton Ings, where you will encounter on the east bank the aptly named 'Asylum' landing. It is now disused, but at one time it served a narrow-gauge railway that took coal to the nearby hospital. The nomenclature is apt since it not only still offers a refuge and strength (just take note of the size of the stone) and a very present help in trouble or out of it but the channel of the river at that bend pursues something of an erratic, if indeed not lunatic, course, quite contrary to the usual laws. Anyone with a craft that is at the 6' limit needs to take extra care when negotiating the area. In addition, everyone needs to keep a careful lookout since it is a popular spot for craft to be moored in such a way that they are successfully camouflaged by the overhanging branches of the bankside growth that is almost lush on the west side.

Next comes Skelton railway bridge (with an overhead cable that does little to draw attention to itself just before it), where you take the port arch, and immediately after it the riverside dwellings with private moorings that go to mark the beginnings of the extremely popular village and pub, the Fox, that are Nether Poppleton. In fact, so busy is the place that it is better known as 'Ever Popularton'. There are pub moorings for visitors, but you may well find

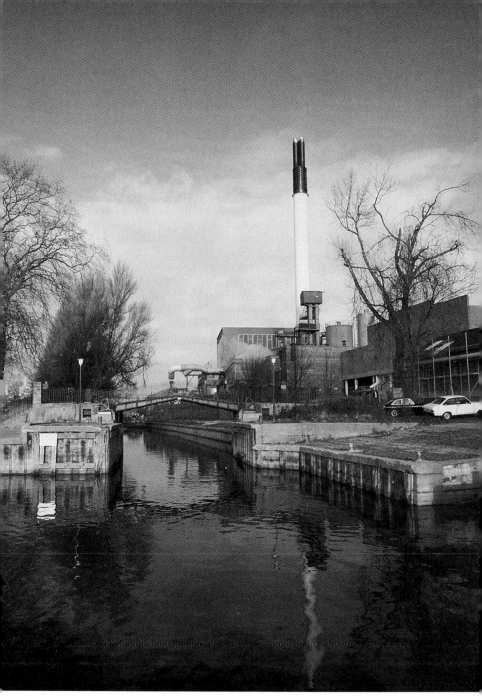

The unmistakable entry to the River Foss in York. Passage through the lock (a few hundred yards upstream in the basin) can only be made after prior arrangement with the river manager at Naburn.

that you need to pass them by and find a quieter spot where you can get your bows to the bank and take the short walk back, so busy is it likely to be. There is one such 'inlet' not far downstream from the pub itself – needless to say, also popular. Sadly, it is not a sensible candidate for anchoring and going ashore by dinghy, since there is a chance that quite a few river cowboys will frequent the area, some in a tanked up state, to test out the planing capabilities of their over-proud prowed vessels.

A couple more miles upstream, with the surrounding scenery improving all the while, lies the village of Beningborough where there is a landing for what Mr. Griffiths (of *East Coast Swatchways*) would call 'shoal craft'. By this time you are deep in some of the best of the countryside so far (with the names of the areas and river stretches telling you so, if you have been unobservant enough to miss it: Ivy Bank, Alder Tree Reach, Bouchier's Scalp). By this time also, the river has narrowed considerably and from here on there are very good, hazardous reasons why you should approach the banks only with the greatest of caution: not only is this where the famous (or notorious or even infamous according to your taste and vocabulary) Clay Huts begin, but there are also many places where piles have rotted and fallen into the river. Both sets of hazards are more often than not indiscernible to the naked eye, so a central course and a wary eye are called for from now on.

However, no wary eye is needed to detect the charms of Nun Monkton Pool and the diminutive village that just overlooks it. It is here that the (sad to say quite unnavigable) River Nidd leaves the Ouse at a sharply right-angled turn to port while the Ouse itself takes an equally sharp turn to starboard; a real 'T' junction marking the parting of the ways. And it certainly is such a parting, for

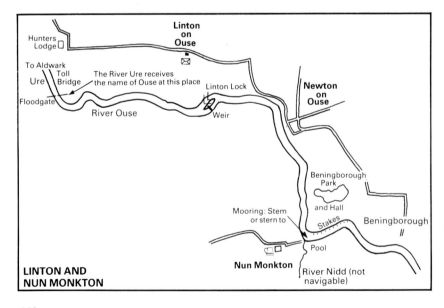

LINTON AND
NUN MONKTON

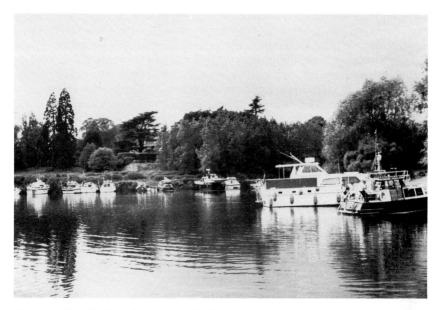

The pool at Nun Monkton: journey's end for *Valcon*, and a truly heavenly haven to heave to in. The River Nidd (not navigable) is to the left of the picture and the Ouse continues upstream to the Ure at centre right.

what was at Trent Falls a mighty waterway, almost a world too wide for the shrunk shanks of any pleasure craft, has now become little more than a substantial stream, calming down and addressing itself to the task of becoming a miniature, which is precisely what it does when it reaches Ouse Gill Beck above the locks at Linton.

Skippers arriving here may have had their share of adversity in the seaway of the Ouse, and some may even have felt that, like the toad, that stretch of the river could be called ugly and venomous; but even if they haven't, they are still likely to appreciate the charms of the pool by Nun Monkton as being something of a jewel in the crown. And while the pool is by no means the head of navigation (that is, except for those who have achieved the spot with 6' draught) nevertheless it is so much a location that possesses so much that is pleasing and so little that is without appeal that surely it must be found in *As You Like It*:

> 'Sweet are the uses of adversity,
> Which, like the toad, ugly and venomous,
> Wears yet a precious jewel in its head:
> And this our life exempt from public haunt
> Finds tongues in trees, books in the running brooks,
> Sermons in stones and good in everything.'

From time to time there is commercial dredging for aggregate here, and it does seem something of an unlikely activity in the midst of what is otherwise almost inactive in its ineffability. If you have moored for only a little time at King's Staithe in York, the chances are that you will have seen the very barge, grab and operators, for that is where most of their catch is discharged.

If you take the turn to the right you will come face to face with an avenue of trees that presents itself like some tunnel through which only the smallest and quietest of craft should be permitted to travel; and it is a more than suitable exit from a village mooring that is not absolutely without facilities, but is, in essence, so removed from the world at large that only a fairy tale brook could be brooked as its symbol.

From here on, if you have a craft of suitable draught, and around three feet is perhaps the optimum, it is roses, roses all the way: Newton upon Ouse; Linton, with its Clay Huts, sandbars, wood and private island; Aldwark with its toll bridge and hostelry; Lower Dunsforth; Swale Nab; Aldborough Roman Landing; Boroughbridge; Littlethorpe; and Ripon. *Valcon* was 'restricted by draught' and so these waters were denied to her; but I was fortunate enough to be piloted from Ripon downstream by the Vice Commodore of the Ripon Motor Boat Club aboard his Thames-built cruiser *Cygnus Verdre*.

From the club's headquarters at Littlethorpe (which they own) the canal runs for just under a mile, in most pleasant rural surroundings, to Oxclose Lock, a small but well kept affair. After the lock, you enter the totally unthreatening waters of the River Ure, and before you get to the next lock at Westwick, there are two items of interest: the Royal Engineers Bridging School at Holbeck on the south bank; and Newby Hall on the north. Then, immediately after the unusually named Arrows Bridge (A1) there are club moorings giving access to the village of Langthorpe with its recent development in mature brick, and the conveniently placed hostelry, the Fox and Hounds.

Next, Boroughbridge is the proud possessor of two 'Marines': the Anchor and the Tower, as well as BWB facilities and those associated with prosperous market towns. Then it is not far to Milby Lock and on to Swale Nab where the River Swale joins in; and most people will then press on again to the next logical and most demanding stopping station, the well-treed bank that gives access to the Bay Horse public house, half a mile below that splendidly famous tollbridge at Aldwark.

Somewhere en route, the river changes its name to Ouse, and it certainly has become that by the time you reach Linton Lock and Newton-upon-Ouse, the two places of major interest before you navigate the avenues of trees I mentioned earlier that guides you into the watery glade that is the pool at Nun Monkton.

For the stretch I have just described (Ripon to Nun Monkton) I can do no better than refer the interested reader to the Ripon Motor Boat Club's excellent guide. This is what they say about the accessibility of their home:

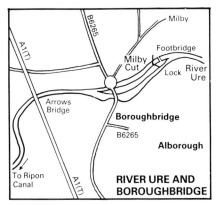

RIVER URE AND BOROUGHBRIDGE

WESTWICK LOCK

Boroughbridge,
North Yorkshire

Restricting dimensions   61' x 16'6"
Rise and fall   10'
Hand operated   •
Boater operated   •
Windlass required   •
Facilities nearby None

OXCLOSE LOCK

Boroughbridge,
North Yorkshire

Restricting dimensions   61' x 16'6"
Rise and fall   12'
Hand operated   •
Boater operated   •
Windlass required   •
Facilities nearby
Ripon 2 miles.

Remarks
Ripon Cathedral – 2 miles.
Superb Cistercian ruins at Fountains Abbey –
5 miles.

MILBY LOCK

Boroughbridge,
North Yorkshire

Restricting dimensions   61' x 16'6"
Rise and fall   10'
Hand operated   •
Boater operated   •
Windlass required   •
Facilities nearby
½ mile Boroughbridge

🐟   In Boroughbridge
🛢   In Boroughbridge
✉   1 mile
⚓   Boroughbridge Sanitary Station
S ⤴   In Boroughbridge
⛽

'Littlethorpe Marina is the home mooring and property of the Ripon Motor Boat Club. The size of vessel that can be accommodated is determined by the profile of the arched bridge a short distance downstream, the depth of water, and the length of the locks. A *Seamaster 30* with navigation lamps etc. removed from the wheel house top so that it requires 8 feet 6 inches of height over 7 feet 9 inches of width can just pass the bridge. 3 feet 6 inches to 3 feet 9 inches is the generally accepted draught limit. The arrangements within the marina preclude the mooring of vessels over 35 feet LOA, but visiting narrow boats up to 60 feet LOA can wind in the marina entrance and moor to the canal bank beside the marina.'

The club is happy to provide overnight moorings for visiting members of other clubs; moorings for longer periods can sometimes be made available by prior arrangement. There is a slipway for trailed craft; and there are water, toilet, waste disposal and car parking facilities. Until recently, the club's HQ was the ship *Enid*, but now they have built a fine clubhouse where visitors are welcome. It is on the phone: (0765) 701751. So; many water miles, light years and atmospheres away from its confluence with the Trent and Humber, here, combining the best of Gill Beck, the Ure, the Swale and the Ripon Canal, can be tasted the real spirit of the Great Yorkshire Ouse. For variety, charm, challenge and charisma, one must journey a long way to find a serious contender for the title.

RIVER URE AND
THE RIPON CANAL

Distances
Ure. Ouse to Oxclose Lock 8 miles
Ripon Canal. Oxclose Lock to Ripon 1 mile
Non-tidal throughout.

Dimensions
Ure
    Length 57'
    Beam 14'6"
    Draught 5' (at very best)
    Air draught 8'6"
Ripon Canal
    Length 57'
    Beam 14'6"
    Draught 3'6"
    Air draught 8'6"

Locks Ure 2; Ripon Canal 1

Traffic
Exclusively light pleasure craft and hand-powered vessels.

Remarks
Shallow (extremely so in parts; beware Clay Huttes!) but just as pretty as it is shallow.
The British Waterways Board is the navigation authority from Swale Nab to Ripon only. Current upstream limit of navigation is Littlethorpe i.e. Ripon Motor Boat Club Marina. The Board's locks at Milby, Westwick and Oxclose are operated by boatmen at all times. Some assistance may be given if the canalmen are present.

O.S. Maps (1:50,000)
    99 Northallerton and Ripon
    100 Malton and Pickering

THE RIVER SWALE

For a vessel not exceeding 1 metre draught, it is possible to get a short way up this offshoot of the Ouse. By exercising caution, the prudent skipper can get about a mile above Myton bridge; and you can moor there, although there is little to tempt many people since the place is remote (without feeling it) and the leg of less than a mile just exposes the village of Myton itself, which is possessed of little that is of interest or appeal. There are hazards en route, apart from the weed and the ever-too-close river bed, in the form of dredging wires, for the stretch is dredged from time to time. All in all, there can be few skippers who would feel it worthwhile taking the risks.

RIVER DERWENT AND POCKLINGTON CANAL

Distances

Derwent. Barmby/Ouse to Stamford Bridge
20 miles

Pocklington. River Derwent, Cottingwith to
Canal Head, Pocklington 10 miles

Non-tidal throughout.

Dimensions

Derwent	Pocklington
Length 55'	Length 55'
Beam 14'	Beam 14'
Draught 4'	Draught 3'
Air draught 10'	Air draught 9'

Locks Derwent 1; Pocklington 9 (but not in
repair)

Traffic

There is only enough water for extremely light
draught craft. At times there can be as little as
one foot of water over some shoal patches; and
when there is flood there can be as little as 5'
headroom. Thus, it is difficult to suggest anything other than to consult the tidal barrage
keepers at Barmby who will advise.

Remarks

Unused, unpredictable, unexploited but by no
means unexceptionable.

Levels in River Derwent may be reduced on a
temporary basis during operation of the
Barmby Barrage by the Yorkshire Water
Authority. Give estimated arrival time to the
attendant at the barrage (Selby ☎ (0757)
638579).

OS Maps (1:50,000)
105 York

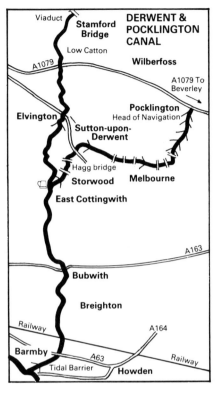

Derwent Boat Certificates may be obtained
from:
The Attendant,
Yorkshire Water Authority,
1 The Bungalows,
Barmby Tidal Barrage,
Barmby-on-the-Marsh,
Goole, York.
☎ Selby (0757) 638579

The River Derwent and the Pocklington Canal

There are hazards in these waterways also; mainly associated with general shal-
lowness (draughts above 5' are not recommended to attempt the navigation at
all, and nothing above 4' should attempt Sutton Lock) and the operation of the
tidal barrage and sluices at Barmby may cause unexpected, unannounced,
wide and rapid variations in the river level. Even upstream of Sutton Lock, the
river is subject to rapid rise and fall depending upon the severity of the recent
rainfall in the catchment area.

It is worth noting that the Yorkshire Water Authority's business here is a massive one; the Derwent drains one tenth of Yorkshire and supplies one sixth of its population with water. The length of the Derwent is 75 miles and with its tributaries it has a catchment area of 722 square miles. Its average recorded flow is 18.3 cubic metres per second, although the maximum recorded flood flow is 124 cubic metres per second – 25 times the dry weather flow. Bearing these figures in mind, it is clear that rise and fall and flow can be major factors for anyone thinking of cruising the river.

Although it is possible to negotiate the waterway with the figures I have quoted above, it can only be done safely if you know exactly where to find, or, more relevantly, to avoid, the rock shoals. In the absence of charts it is wise to accept a maximum draught for the river as three feet; and if you are in any doubt at all, a telephone call to the barrage keeper should set your mind at rest.

The river and the canal are both charming waterways, and local fans are doing all they can to ensure they are brought into, and kept in, a state that they deserve. They occupy one of the prettiest parts of Yorkshire and are well worth visiting for a couple of days, or weeks, if you have a suitable craft. Anyone seriously thinking of trying the river or the canal should obtain copies of the guides to the river, published by the Yorkshire Derwent Trust, and to the canal, published by the Pocklington Canal Amenity Society, details of which may be found under 'Recommended Reading'.

The Yorkshire Water Authority takes its leisure responsibilities seriously and has published a set of *Notes for River Derwent Boat Users*. The following have been extracted from those notes:

'The discharge of the lowest reach of the River Derwent is controlled by a pair of sluice gates at Barmby tidal barrage close to the confluence with the Ouse, and the tide is normally excluded from the Derwent. Notwithstanding this control, the level of the Derwent fluctuates by varying amounts depending on the fresh water discharge in the river, tidal conditions in the Ouse and the distance from the barrage. On occasions, such as when a high fresh flow in the Ouse coincides with a high spring tide, the gates are opened to allow the tide into the Derwent. On other occasions, the gates are specially opened to reduce the level. Boat users are accordingly advised to take the same precautions when navigating or mooring as on a tidal river. The Yorkshire Water Authority cannot accept responsibility for any claims arising from damage to vessels.

The sluice gate control system at the barrage normally operates to maintain a certain level in the river except when, to facilitate land drainage, a free discharge is permitted at the barrage. Boat users are therefore advised to proceed with caution as they may encounter localised shallow spots or shoals in the river channel.

The floating landing stage 200m upstream of the barrage is intended purely for the use of boat users waiting to use the lock or using the toilets or toilet disposal facilities provided adjacent to the landing stage. Mooring for any other purpose or for a long period of time is not permitted, and can be dangerous due to the fluctuating water levels in the river at this point. Boat users wishing to use the lock should moor at the appropriate place provided either in the River Ouse or the River Derwent, and summon the attendant by means of the bell provided at the side of the lock. UNDER NO CIRCUMSTANCES SHOULD BOAT USERS ATTEMPT TO OPERATE THE LOCK THEMSELVES.

Boating

The Derwent provides attractive water for boats. From Barmby Barrage up to Sutton Lock it was fully tidal till 1975. The lock at Sutton has been restored by volunteers, who are now working on locks farther up river. Stamford Bridge can be reached by boats entering at Barmby from the Ouse; the reaches above Stamford Bridge also provide boating water.

Many boat owners moor their craft at points along the river.

Please:

Do not interfere with moored boats or with mooring ropes.

Do not trespass on a moored boat to fish from it or for any other reason.

Immediately report any drifting boat to the Y.W.A. lock-keeper at Barmby telephone Selby (07578) 638579.

Boat users – Keep a proper lookout when on the move.

Watch your choice of moorings and avoid mooring at a nature reserve.

Do not moor where you will create a nuisance or hazard to other users of the river or users of the lands adjoining.

Moor securely. The water level of the river fluctuates widely; allow for this when mooring up.

Lock up your boat when leaving it for any length of time.

Keep your moorings clean and tidy.

Use locks and apparatus in the proper manner.

Sutton Lock

There is no navigation authority for the River Derwent. It is generally accepted that there is a public right of navigation on the former tidal length of the Derwent between the River Ouse and Sutton, but conflicting views on the legal status of navigation on the river upstream of that point have been recorded.

The Authority stands neutral on that matter but, as owner of the structure and the upper or guillotine gate of Sutton Lock, allows their use on the terms described below. Ownership of the lower gates rests with the Yorkshire Derwent Trust Ltd.

No assurance can be given as to the continued availability of the lock should damage, deterioration or operational needs prevent its safe use. Among these needs is the practice during the early and late months of each year of propping open the lower gates so as to pass floodwater and scour out deposits of silt and sand at the tail of the lock.

In the interests of safety and water conservation the guillotine gate and the windlass are kept padlocked. The Authority will give keys to the holders of Derwent Boat Certificates on the following terms:-

a. The same key will work both padlocks, which are not intended to be changed for at least one year.

b. Keys are not transferable.

c. Applicants for keys are required to sign an undertaking as to the proper operation of the lock in the way described below.

d. Requests for keys should be made on the appropriate form. The applicant must hold a current Derwent Boat Certificate, or must apply for one at the same time.

Please note that the 'life' of the keys will depend on two things: first, the padlocks not being removed or damaged and secondly, the keys or duplicates of them not coming into the possession of persons who do not hold Derwent Boat Certificates.

Operating Instructions

1. The lock may be used during the hours of daylight only.
2. Use of the lock for canoes and other small inflatable craft, whether powered or not, is not allowed under normal circumstances.
3. On entering the lock craft must be adequately secured or otherwise controlled as a precaution against turbulence in the chamber.
4. The gate paddles must not be operated until the gates are closed.
5. A special windlass, kept locked in the box near to the chamber, operates the paddle for the guillotine gate. Access to crank the paddle is from the towpath on the west side of the lock. The windlass must be removed from the spindle immediately after use, and returned to its box. The box must be left locked.
6. No attempt must be made to open or close the gates by any other means, or before the water levels on each side of the gate are equal.

7. The mechanism for lifting the guillotine gate is on the island side of the chamber. The gearing of the two spindles differs – the one nearest to the tail of the lock being lower geared than the other.

8. After leaving the chamber it is essential that
   a. The paddles are closed
   b. The guillotine gate is padlocked in the closed position, and
   c. The lower gates are left open, contrary to normal waterway practice.

9. Please note that the occupant of the cottage on the island is not a lock-keeper, nor is he employed by the Water Authority in any capacity. Cases of emergency should be reported to the Authority's attendant at Barmby Tidal Barrage, Barmby-on-the-Marsh, Goole. (Telephone Selby (0757) 638579).

10. There is no right of access along the footway crossing the weirs on the main river.

11. No boats may be moored within 25 metres of the entrance to the fish pass adjacent to the lock, nor in any way so as to obstruct the entrance to the pass.

12. A temporary mooring facility, together with a sullage disposal room and water supply, is available on the east bank of the river just upstream of Elvington road bridge. A standard British Waterways Board lock is fitted to the door.

13. Boat users upstream of Sutton Lock are requested to note that, under certain circumstances, the functioning of Elvington Sluices may result in a rapid lowering of river level without warning.

BARMBY LOCK

The Attendant,
Yorkshire Water Authority,
1 The Bungalows,
Barmby Tidal Barrage,
Barmby-on-the-Marsh,
Goole,
York
☎ Selby (0757) 638579

Restricting dimensions 65' x 16'6"
Rise and fall Varies – see special remarks. Owners of vessels with a draught exceeding 5' are advised not to enter the Derwent.

Mechanised ● Remotely operated radial sector gates.
Keeper operated ● Summon attendant by bell at side of lock.

Facilities nearby
⚓ 🚽
🅆🅒 Toilet waste disposal facility
🗔 ✉ ♪ S
in village – but see note on mooring at lock below.

Remarks
See page 214. *Notes for Derwent Boat Users.*

SUTTON OR ELVINGTON LOCK

Restricting dimensions 60' x 14'.
Rise and fall Varies – see special remarks.
Mechanised ● Guillotine gate secured by pad lock.
Hand operated ● Keys available f.o.c. to Derwent Boat Certificate holders. See operat ing instructions .
Boater operated ●
Windlass required ● Special windlass provided – secured in box at lockside (key also required).
Facilities nearby
⚓ 🚽
🅆🅒 Toilet waste disposal facility
🗔 ✉ ♪ S
in Sutton/Elvington – please do not leave craft moored so as to prevent use of waste disposal point.

EAST COTTINGWITH LOCK

BWB
East Cottingwith Lock,
East Cottingwith,
York

Restricting dimensions   75' x 10'
Rise and fall   8'
Hand operated   ●
Boater operated   ●
Windlass required   ●
Facilities nearby

🍺   Kings Head – 400 yards
S   General store – 400 yards
✉   400 yards
☏   400 yards

SWING BRIDGE NO. 1

BWB,
Storwood,
East Cottingwith,
York

Restricting dimensions   Width 10' gutway
Hand operated   ●
Boater operated   ●
Facilities nearby None

SWING BRIDGE NO. 2

Restricting dimensions   Width 10' gutway
Hand operated   ●
Boater operated   ●
Facilities nearby None

Remarks
Access is across private land.

SWING BRIDGE NO. 3
(GARDHAM LOCK)

BWB
Melbourne,
York

Restricting dimensions   75' x 10'
Rise and fall   5'
Hand operated   ●
Boater operated   ●
Facilities nearby None

Remarks
Access to lock over private land. BWB access only.

GARDHAM LOCK

BWB,
Gardham Lock,
Melbourne,
York

Restricting dimensions   75' x 10'
Rise and fall   5' approx.
Hand operated   ●
Boater operated   ●
Windlass required   ●
Facilities nearby None

Remarks
Access to lock is over private land. BWB access only.

SWING BRIDGE NO. 4

Restricting dimensions   Width 10' gutway
Hand operated   ●
Boater operated   ●
Facilities nearby None

Remarks
Access is across private land.

FIXED BRIDGE No. 5

Restricting dimensions   10' gutway
Hand operated   ●
Boater operated   ●
Facilities nearby None

VI. THE RIVERS ANCHOLME AND HULL via the River Humber

I first encountered the River Humber by way of its five-mile-wide estuary mouth some years ago on a flat-calm sea in a flat-thick fog. I managed to navigate my way across by a combination of stereophonic listening to try to ensure keeping mid-way between the easily distinguishable tones of the fog signals; by the ritualistic crossing of fingers ('By the pricking of my thumbs, something wicked this way comes '); and by the regular applications of spirituous liquors to the troubled parts for the relief of me and my sore psyche. As a result of that initial experience, I have always held the Humber in a very special kind of esteem – if not indeed plain, old-fashioned awe.

Nor am I alone in contemplating the river in that way. Since my foggy crossing, I have met hundreds of skippers who have been more than eloquent about the Humber but whose opinions have been pretty well equally divided, and usually extreme. One group perceives it as a river that is neither to be cruised nor explored just for the sake of doing so, but rather as a mighty tideway that should only be used, cautiously and soberly, as a necesary passage route for safer and better waters. The other group takes a diametrically opposed position: the Humber is an intriguing and altogether pleasing river that offers more than ample grounds for racing, sailing, cruising or just pottering about from place to place, calling at every marina, haven, creek and anchorage. I can see both points of view; and, nailing my colours to the mast, must confess that I would dearly like to spend a couple of seasons on the river, since it offers so many opportunities, combinations, challenges and pleasures within its forty muddy miles from Trent Falls to Spurn.

The approaches from seaward, whether from north or south, will be aimed at picking up Spurn light float and/or Spurn light house. From the south, there are three areas to be avoided when coming up from (say) Great Yarmouth or The Wash, and they are the DZ zone, Rosse Spit and Haile Sand; and from the north (Bridlington or Scarborough) there is just one: the Binks. A course of five miles off, from both directions, avoids all hazards.

There are only two approaches from inland: from the Trent, perhaps the anchorage by Trent Falls as a waiting-over spot, or from the Yorkshire Ouse, perhaps from Blacktoft Jetty, if you have a sturdy vessel and can afford the fees. From either place, the demarkation symbol of the Apex light reminds you that there is in fact a choice of two ways to go (it can hardly be said that there are two channels although from time to time that is the case). The main big-ship channel is on the Lincolnshire (south) side, although the channels vary dramatically in the Humber as the sketch map shows. There is however, an entirely different kind of channel on the other side: just over a mile from Apex, and giving access to the diminutive settlements of Faxfleet and Broomfleet,

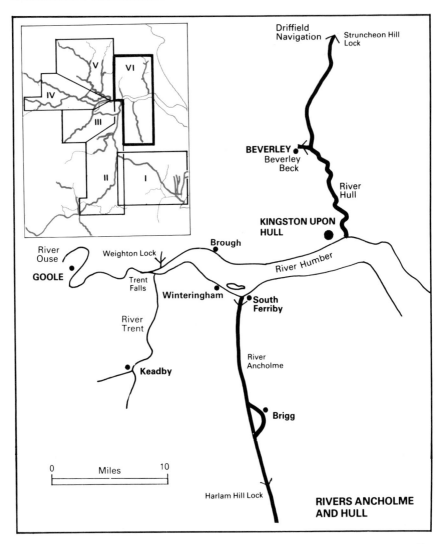

there is to be found the entrance to the Market Weighton Canal; never really completed and now almost unused. The lock is difficult to approach from the river because of the proximity of the ever-changing sandbanks in a part of the river that is no longer traversed by craft drawing more than a metre or so. At the time of writing, the Associated British Ports *Humber chart* shows a drying bar by the Faxfleetness entrance and a half metre bar from the east, but with a 'waiting' pool just outside the lock with a depth of 1.8m. In passing, it is interesting to note that South Ferriby also possesses such a 'hole', but with more water at 2.7m. In addition, the canal may be used for sluicing off the land

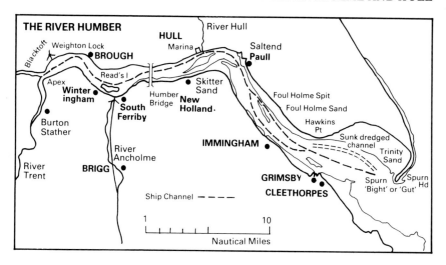

NAVIGATION AUTHORITIES

The River Ancholme

Anglian Water,
Waterside House,
Waterside North,
Lincoln LN2 5HA
☎ (0522) 25231

AW office and lock-keeper,
South Ferriby
VHF channel 16, 06, 10, 12, 14
☎ Barton (0652) 635219

Northern Area Office,
Guy Gibson Hall,
Manby Park,
Louth LN11 8UR
☎ (050 782) 8101

Southern Area Office,
Aqua House,
Harvey Street,
Lincoln LN1 1TF
☎ (0522) 39221

The River Humber

Associated British Ports ,
Harbour master,
Kingston House Tower,
Bond St,
Hull HU1 3ER
☎ (0482) 27171

The River Hull

Navigation authority
Hull City Council,
Engineer's Department,
Guildhall,
Alfred Gelder Street,
Hull HU1 2AA
☎ (0482) 223111

Harbour master,
Drypool Bridge
☎ (0482) 222287
VHF channels 16 and 12 for three hours before
and one hour after HW.

VHF channel 6 is reserved for ship use on
Saturday mornings irrespective of tide times.

Water authority
Yorkshire Water Authority
Rivers Division,
21 Park Square South,
Leeds LS1 2QG
☎ (0532) 440191

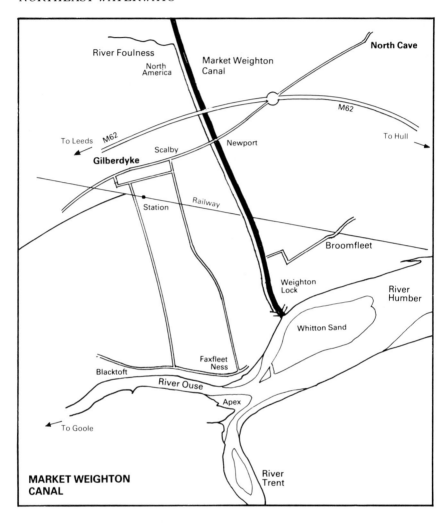

MARKET WEIGHTON CANAL

WEIGHTON OR HUMBER LOCK

Yorkshire Water Authority,
Rivers Division,
21 Park Square South,
Leeds LS1 2QG
☎ (0532) 430191

Restricting dimensions   66′ x 14′9″
Rise and fall Sea lock -varies. Craft of approx.
4′0″ max.draught may pass.

Keeper operated   ● Use of lock possible by special prior arrangement only – details from Rivers Division, above.
Lock-keeper ☎ (0430) 41122

Remarks
No YWA moorings available for public use. (These mooring facilities at locks and toilet waste disposal points are provided for temporary use only.)

and will then be, of course, impossible to enter. If however, in spite of all the drawbacks, you still harbour a yen to pen into the quaint and remote and have a boat with no more draught than one metre, you should negotiate your visit through the Yorkshire Water Authority who have restored the mechanics to full working order without destroying in any way their charming, ancient visage.

Once inside the locked waterway, you really are in backwoods territory. There are some small communities around, but they are very small and none of them is very close. The nearest is Broomfleet on Broomfleet Island where there is a pub and a shop; and then there are Faxfleet and Blacktoft, and upstream Newport and Gilberdyke.

The navigation is straight and much used by fishermen, for whom the YWA has co-operatively arranged for it to be well served. There is little for the tourist cruising man to see or to contemplate and this waterway must be looked on as one of the most remote, unvisited and quaint of canals, although interesting enough for those who have the passion for history. Otherwise, it is the haven of the lock that must be the main attraction for those who are looking for a staging post while on passage to further parts. The YWA is now the navigation authority and has got out some brief notes for the guidance of those who have in mind to use the canal. They are as follows:

Boating

1. Observe a maximum speed of 5mph, or such speed that is insufficient to create a breaking wash (whichever is the lesser).
2. Observe permitted hours of passage over match fishing lengths – do not pass beyond a red flag.
3. No boat should advance beyond the River Foulness junction with the canal during the months of April-June (inclusive).
4. When passing anglers and moored craft, reduce speed and avoid the shallow waters at the canal bank.
5. Do not moor where you will create a nuisance or hazard to other users of the canal or users of the lands adjoining. Moor at designated landing places whenever possible.
6. Sea toilets should be sealed throughout the canal to avoid problems of pollution.

Wildlife

All visitors to the canal should endeavour to avoid disturbing the birds and other animal life along the banks. Do not pick or uproot flowers or plants or unnecessarily trample canalside vegetation.

Mutual Tolerance

Respect the other users' activities. Exercise the greatest possible courtesy and toleration. With consideration, all parties can enjoy their particular interest without conflict.

Annual boat licences are issued free on application to the: Yorkshire Water Authority Rivers Division, 21 Park Square South, Leeds LS1 2QG. ☎ (0532) 440191.

The Market Weighton Canal Society is keen for craft to visit. Please contact G. B. Miles, Acting Secretary, M.W.C.S., 47 Market Place, Market Weighton, York, YO4 3AJ. ☎ York (0696) 72740.

The ruling dimensions are as follows:
Length: 66′
Beam: 14′
Draught: 4′
Air Draught: 9′ at lowest bridge: A63 (for information re stop-over facilities, contact YWA office: the bridge within the lock area demands prior consultation).
Lock-keeper ☎ (0430) 41122. .

N.B: The Cruising Guide issued by the Ripon Motor Boat Club gives excellent guidance for those with a wish and a will to proceed to Sod House Lock!

Because of some of the problematic aspects of the approach to this waterway, and what must be deemed its marginal appeal except to enthusiasts with special causes to plead, most skippers will tend towards the Lincolnshire coast down to Whitton Hill, past the West and East Dyke lights (Nos 42 and 40) where there is a useful anchorage 200 yards downstream of the 42 light, safely inshore of it. 'Safely' meaning here, well out of the shipping lane and in good water and holding ground. Anchor signals and watches needed!

Off the village of Whitton itself which from time to time exhibits a pretty façade to the river is the first of the 'floats', those navigational aids for which the Humber is rightly well known. At one time, they were manned (the mind boggles at the concept) but now they are automatic. In spite of the colour of some of them, they still remind me, like the Roaring Middle in The Wash, of a banana boat. But seriously, they, and all the other navigational aids, beacons, boards, lights, daymarks and so on, are impeccably maintained and together with the charts and notices to mariners issued by ABP Humber, offer a faultless guide to all who navigate the area. The following notice gives some idea of the formidability of the task involved:

NOTICE TO MARINERS (No. H.69/1984)
NEW HOLLAND CHANNEL MIDDLE HUMBER
MARINERS ARE WARNED that a survey of the New Holland Channel carried out on 3rd July, 1984 shows that shoal patches with drying heights of 0.1 metres above chart datum exist close to the ships course in the vicinity of No. 20A light buoy.
    MARINERS ARE FURTHER WARNED that rapid changes are taking place in this channel and navigation should be carried out with caution.
(G. SMITH: HARBOUR MASTER. HUMBER)

The first proper 'havens-of-call' are Brough and Winteringham, facing one another across the two miles of the breadth of the river. I have been fortunate to have been shown some of the intricacies of the two havens and many more of the river itself by Mel Parish, the mate of the century-old Humber Yawl Club whose headquarters and clubhouse are at Brough, where you will be made exceedingly welcome by the hosts of their lively membership. Entries to these two havens are constantly changing, but the two sketches give some idea of the trickiness that awaits strangers; it must be well worthwhile to contact the Humber Yawl Club, telephone: Hull (0482) 667224 and/or visit shoresides well ahead of your proposed trip. Tides need careful consideration and, although the club is indeed hospitable, they do not have enough 'free' moorings to be able to house a chance arrival. For craft drawing no more than 4'6" (1½ metres) access to both havens is restricted to $-2/+1½$ hours high water.

TABLE OF DISTANCES

	Spurn Head	Grimsby	Hull	Beverley	South Ferriby	Brigg	Brandy Wharf	Brough	Market Weighton Lock	Trent Falls
Spurn Head		6	22	32	28	38	43	33	35	37
Grimsby	6		16	26	22	32	37	27	29	31
Hull	22	16		10	6	16	21	11	13	15
Beverley	32	26	10		16	26	31	21	23	25
South Ferriby	28	22	6	16		10	15	5	7	9
Brigg	38	32	16	26	10		5	15	17	19
Brandy Wharf	43	37	21	31	15	5		20	22	24
Brough	33	27	11	21	5	15	20		2	4
Market Weighton Lock	35	29	13	23	7	17	22	2		2
Trent Falls	37	31	15	25	9	19	24	4	2	

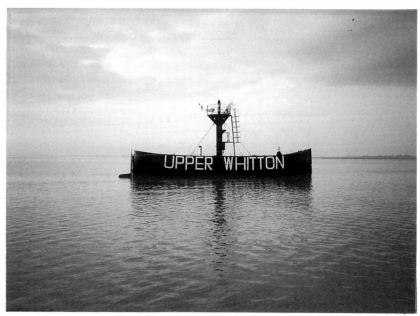

Upper Whitton light float – the first on the Humber.

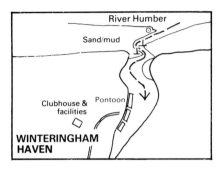

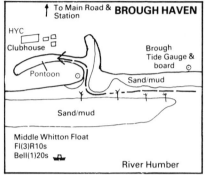

Not far away from Brough and on the other side of the river is Read's Island (for me, notorious since I was often shown the bleak spot as a child, usually with threats of abandonment to its rat-infested wastes if I did not 'behave'). When I called there in 1984, the island itself was the subject of Notice to Mariners No. H.84/1984. 'NOTICE IS HEREBY GIVEN that considerable erosion is taking place along the north side of Read's Island in the Upper Humber and the floodbanks are being affected.' Just another example of the ever-changing aspect of the Humber; and quite a few locals told me they were expecting 'almost any day now' that the river would change its channels and once more come on the south side of the island.

The main attraction of the island for any cruising man must be its well protected channel by the Lincolnshire bank, being the one that gives access to the lock at Ferriby Sluice, and then to the hinterland via the River Ancholme. The entrance to the approach haven is made obvious by the towering cement factory, and there is little danger of missing it. Legend, aided and abetted by 'local experts' who are not really local nor indeed expert at anything at all but the con-

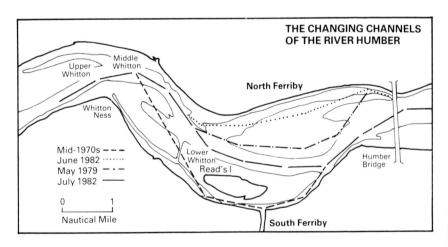

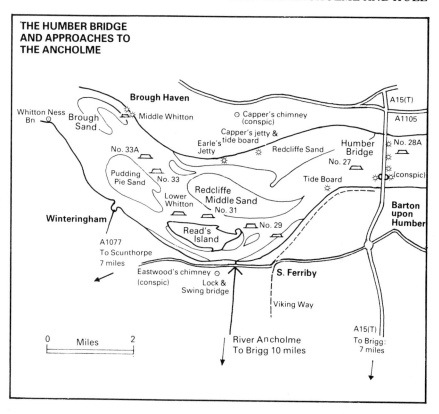

THE HUMBER BRIDGE
AND APPROACHES TO
THE ANCHOLME

Brough Haven

Whitton Ness
Bn

Brough
Sand

Middle Whitton

Capper's chimney
(conspic)

A15(T)

A1105

Capper's jetty &
tide board

Earle's
Jetty

No. 33A

Redcliffe Sand

Humber
Bridge

No. 28A

No. 27

(conspic)

Pudding
Pie Sand

No. 33

Lower
Whitton

Redcliffe
Middle Sand

No. 31

Tide Board

Barton
upon
Humber

Winteringham

No. 29

Read's
Island

A1077
To Scunthorpe
7 miles

Eastwood's chimney
(conspic)

Lock &
Swing bridge

S. Ferriby

Viking Way

A15(T)

0   Miles   2

River Ancholme
To Brigg 10 miles

To Brigg:
7 miles

sumption of the local ample ale, has it that there is always a fathom in the south
channel by the island – whether you use the east or the west approach – and that
it runs for the full length. However, a considered reading of the ABP chart, and
a consultation with any of those skippers who actually and regularly use the
channel, will recommend a high-water passage from the eastern entrance, leaving the main shipping channel of the Humber at No. 32 float (Fl.R.2s) and
then keeping about a cable from the south bank.

The configuration of the haven is such that the shoulders of mud and sand
spits cause something of a double hazard: firstly, they need to be avoided on
their own account, thus dictating a guarded approach, fully opening up the
haven and then making the run in the 'channel' shown in the chartlet (roughly
southeasterly); secondly, just outside in the river there is quite a whirling eddy
so careful attention to the helm and controlled use of power is essential, particularly at times of big spring tides when the rate can get up to 8 knots. The
lock haven does give almost immediately onto the river, so such a precaution
is necessary if you are not to risk ending up on one of the mud mounds that
stand guard over pit and pool.

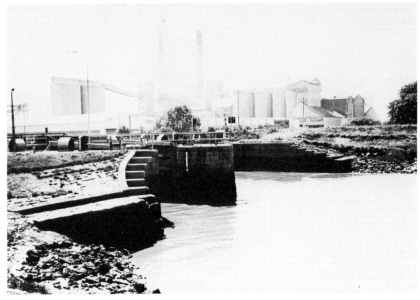

The approach from the River Humber to the lock and sluice at South Ferriby.

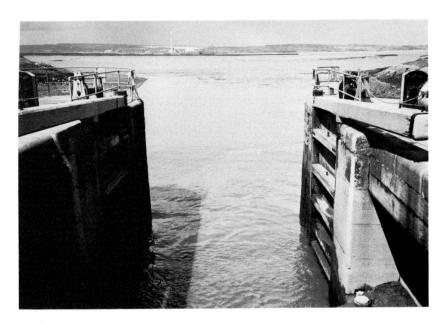

North Ferriby, clearly indicated by the tall chimney, across the river; seen from the lock gates at South Ferriby.

The lock-keepers are on watch from 0700 to 1600, and at other times by arrangement.

I have a very soft spot for the tiny stretch of shoresides that embraces Winteringham Ings, Ferriby Sluice and South Ferriby. Although the cement factory dominates everything in the area (physically that is, for these are people who belong to the old Lincolnshire yellow belly tradition, and nothing, not even the weight of the nomenclature of South Humberside, can daunt them spiritually) there are all kinds of treasures to be found in its shadow. For example, the view from the road bridge, over the lock and across to Read's Island, the River Humber and on to the north bank is one of interest at almost all times. In the morning or evening mists it can achieve vista of quite eerie grandeur, prompting the imagination into all kinds of flights of fancy.

Fancies can also be prompted by the brew offered up by the landlord of the Hope and Anchor; and this hostelry enjoys much of the view I have just described. In *The Tidal Havens of the Wash and Humber* Henry Irving has this to say: 'The saving grace of the place as far as après-sail activities are concerned, is the Hope and Anchor, a basic and spacious public house with good beer, a friendly clientele and a landlord with a keen interest in boats.'

SOUTH FERRIBY
Trent Falls 9 miles
Brigg 10 miles
Moorings
AW just through the lock gates in the River Ancholme; by Clapsons Boatyard a little farther on. Both on the east side of the river.

Marina
AW Office and lock-keeper: ☎ Barton (0652) 635219. There is no marina as such, but the boatyard comes very close.
Clapsons are equipped with VHF Marine. They work Channel 'M', and the call sign is *South Ferriby Base*.

Boatyard
Clapsons ☎ Barton (0652) 635620.
This is an extremely efficiently and happily run place, where you will find much more boating (including sea-going) gear than you might expect.

Club
The nearest thing to a club is the Hope & Anchor pub across the main road.

Facilities
Petrol, shop and post office are in the village which is only a short walk away.

⬥ ● ⚓ ⌒ ✉ S ✕ ▱ 🛒

Remarks
Watch out when making an entry for the mud spits on the shoulders of the haven, and for the strong eddies around the same area. There is a small cut running just to the east of the haven entrance; the berths in there are all private and the manoeuvring called for make it an impossible place for any visitor.

Don't miss the shop in the village: even if you don't need anything make an excuse to visit it – they belong to a tribe that is hardly with us any more . . . and they know the meaning of the word 'service'.

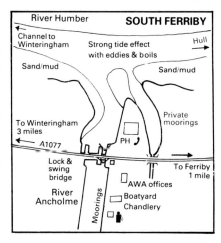

Map: River Humber — SOUTH FERRIBY. Channel to Winteringham. Strong tide effect with eddies & boils. Hull. Sand/mud. Sand/mud. Private moorings. To Winteringham 3 miles. A1077. PH. Lock & swing bridge. River Ancholme. Moorings. AWA offices. To Ferriby 1 mile. Boatyard. Chandlery.

229

Indeed, there is quite a lot to prompt the imagination to work once you start looking around Ferriby Sluice. Those two famous vessels of the Humber Keel Preservation Society, the *Amy Howson* and the *Comrade*, operate from here and they are now being lovingly kept at it to enjoy what must be a totally unexpected rejuvenation. There are also two other burning topics of conjecture, and on occasion, controversy: one is of great long standing, while the other is of more recent origin. The former concerns the quantity and quality of those precipitations that are to be found in the atmosphere resulting (all the locals claim) from the workings at the cement factory. I have been told on more than one occasion that they attack the eyeballs and throats of all humans in the area as well the hulls, brightwork and glazing of all boats. Certainly, after only a brief stop-over, I had a tough time cleansing *Valcon's* wheelhouse in a positive marathon of descaling. The latter and more recent topic is the AWA Aeration Project, known locally as The Bubble, which evenly disperses the salt water from the Humber that comes through with every penning, and so prevents it from proceeding upstream in bulk or just sitting there like a solid wall. The bubbles rise in a controlled manner from the bed of the river in a scheme, apparently working well, of which the authority, in a quiet way, is fairly proud. It is sound ecology; in spite of all local gossip suggesting that it is either a de-pollutant for hazardous 'heavy' water, or an improving sauna for effete fish.

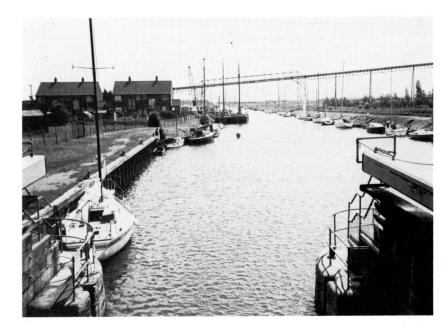

The River Ancholme is a popular one, and nowhere is more popular to moor than the riverside at South Ferriby . . . no matter which side you try first.

SOUTH FERRIBY LOCK

Anglian Water,
Lincoln Division,
South Ferriby Lock,
South Ferriby,
Barton on Humber,
South Humberside
☎ (0652) 635219
VHF channels 16:06, 10, 12, 14
(possibly 74 and 'M' in future). 1 fixed, 2 mobile sets.

Restricting dimensions
Length
a. 68' for 'normal' boat
b. 72' for 'narrow' boat
c. 83' for when 'on a level'
Width
a. 19'10" at top
b. 19'6" halfway
c. 18' at bottom
Draught
Varies from 0' to 26' on the Humber side, being tidal; on the Ancholme side there is no problem on the lower reach for craft drawing 6'+.
Rise and fall Tidal
Hand operated •
Keeper operated •
Facilities nearby
⚓ Tap located near to lock on freshwater side
🛒 🍴 Clapsons Marina nearby

🍺 Hope and Anchor adjacent

S ✉ small grocery store in S. Ferriby village about 1 mile

🍴 About 300 yards towards S. Ferriby or at Hope & Anchor P.H.

Remarks
a. Lock can be used four hours either side of the high tide, but large spring tides of over 22' will involve a delay of up to one hour at high tide.
b. Temporary moorings available adjacent to lock.
c. Short stay permit required for boats not registered with Anglian Water (the navigation authority). Tariff varies according to size of boat.
d. An overhead conveyor is located approximately 300 yards upstream of the lock. At normal river level its height is 40-48' above water level. Very large sailing boats may need to dismast in order to pass by.
e. The River Ancholme is held at normal navigation level between 1 April and 31 October. The remainder of the the time it is at winter level which is approximately 1' lower than summer level. Boatsmen are advised that the river is a land-drainage channel and large fluctuations in level may occur at any time of the year according to prevailing weather conditions.

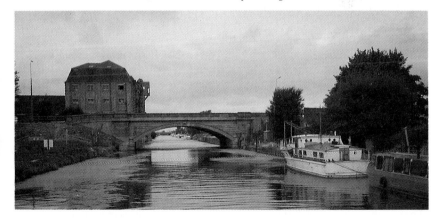

The River Ancholme above the two road bridges in Brigg. Life seldom gets hectic in these parts – although the weed does thrive extremely well.

RIVER ANCHOLME

Distances
South Ferriby (Humber) to Brandy Wharf
(Brandywath) 15 miles
Non-tidal

Dimensions
Length 80'
Beam 19'
Draught 6' to Brigg; then gradually less
Air draught 11'
Lock dimensions
Ferriby 80' x 19' x 6''
Harlam Hill 69' x 16' x 3'

Locks 2

Traffic
Pleasure craft: mainly cruising vessels, with
some sailing (including the *Comrade* and the
Amy Howson Old Timers at South Ferriby).

Remarks
One of the prettiest of the Lincs/Yorks 'flat ter-
rain' rivers: certainly one for 'down the river on
a Sunday afternoon' – especially for those with
young families and even dogs.

OS Map (1:50,000)
112 Scunthorpe

Rase-Ancholme Navigation Trust
c/o Membership Secretary,
Ian N Horsley,
The Anchor Inn,
Brandy Wharf,
Waddingham,
Near Gainsborough,
Lincs.
☎ North Kelsey (065 27) 364

Realities are also well looked after here. The lock-keepers form a very
friendly but not effervescent team, and will see you as right as they can. It is a
good idea on this tidal entry to make sure you have a word with them prior to
visiting: courtesy, common sense and caution regarding the particular conditions being more than enough justification for a telephone call. The AWA has
brought about some excellent improvements at this lock: the provision of
handholds within the lock pit; the installation of a metal access ladder on the
seaward side; and VHF marine radio channels.

Another reality is the facility offered by Clapson's Boatyard. Here you will
find virtually all that you are likely to need, whatever your interest in boating
might be, for they cater for all ages, tastes and all manner of craft. True, there
is no general shop in the immediate vicinity of the lock or boatyard, but there
is such a treasure of a place at the end of a mile walk into the village of South
Ferriby that the lack is almost a virtue. Once inside the classic 'village shop',
it is not quite so easy to decide whether you are still in the realm of fancy or reality; for they combine the nostalgic charm of last century's best habits of 'trade'
(including some assortments of goods that I for one never expected to see
again, having thought they had gone out with my childhood) with an unmistakeably contemporary eye for what makes things tick in South Humberside in
the 1980s. It is a thoroughly refreshing place to visit and you will find that they
can provide you with almost everything a cruising skipper could ask for in the
domestic/victuals line.

Once having prised oneself away from the charms of Ferriby Sluice and its
adjacent village, the next adventure is an expedition south towards Brandy
Wharf. The 'old' and 'new' Ancholme rivers march hand-in-glove towards
Brigg, where are to be found the well-cultivated moorings and discreetly
guarded headquarters of the (almost ancient but certainly honourable) Glanford Boat Club. It is a ten mile trip from Ferriby to Brigg, consisting mainly

of a dead straight course with a succession of bridges that permit passage to craft of 12′ beam at 15′ air draught; that is, all but the very last one just before Brigg, and that restricts your craft to 14′ but it is possible to moor on the downstream side of it and walk into the small market town that is the eponymous subject of Delius's *Brigg Fair*.

For such a straight waterway, the Ancholme offers many surprising delights to the eyes: actual hills, vales, dales, woods and copses that are all scenic and visibly so to the naked eye without it having to be taken to the highest point of the boat in order to perceive anything different from steep and boringly muddy banks. In addition, there are of course, in plain view on some of those plain banks, the usual ration of almost-grazing, immobile fishermen and almost-immobile, grazing cattle.

The moorings by the clubhouse are kept in excellent fettle by the local boating fraternity and you will be made extremely welcome. (Glanford Boat Club, telephone: Brigg (0652) 53412.) The charms of Brigg are not quite what they were when it was a focal point for the thriving farming community that surrounded it, but the chimney of the sugar beet factory still stands, not at ten to three, but ready to spout its sickly sweet odours over the whole neighbourhood whenever the season is on. Fortunately, there is little overlap between the beet season and the cruising season except for those boating fanatics who try to steal an extra month out of the year's calendar. From the victualling point of view, there is not much that you will have to forego as a result of shopping in Brigg; and it still bears the stamp of days gone by, especially near the bridge by the market place.

I knew the Ancholme very well many years ago when I was a seven-year prisoner at the Boys' Grammar School; being instructed, and not at all through gentle persuasion, that I was generally idle, without imagination, couldn't write and should have absolutely nothing to do with the theatre. However, towards my last years at the wretched place, the banks of the Ancholme had provided a lunchtime haven for the three or four of us who would suffer inhaling the noisome fumes from the sugar beet factory so that we could be free to inhale the noxious (but oh, so heady) smoke of illicit cigarettes. That ritual was usually in the company of an equal number of aiding and abetting, but nevertheless not always pliant or yielding, females; refugees from the nearby convent, also a victim of progress and so no more.

(Actually, it wasn't the River Ancholme at all; it was the canal stretch built by French prisoners during the Napoleonic wars but that only makes it all the more poignant.)

With 6′ draught, you will experience no difficulty up to this point, but for those wishing to go to the head of the navigation, no more than 3′ draught is best. There is no sudden falling off in the depth, but it does gradually lose water all along the way, as well as gaining in presence of weed. The locality gets even better as you move upstream and the positive sanctuary of Brandy Wharf (alas no brandy, and certainly none of the illicit stuff, but plenty of nectar-like cider) offers a mooring that shows off some of the best of Lincolnshire's flat appeal. It is also an area that is dyed deep in the wool of our history but very little exploited by archaeologists or historians; indeed, for anyone who has in mind to undertake original research, this must be a prime contender.

All in all, the Ancholme must rank as one of the quietest, most pleasing and non-aggravating cruising rivers in the country; it is possessed of many joys and possesses no serious threat of any kind and there are few waterways about which one can say that.

Certainly the River Humber is not one of them; so it is with proper caution that we cross in order to get to the other river, the River Hull. It is no more than a matter of minutes from Ferriby Sluice to Kingston-upon-Hull, but in those minutes there is much to marvel at: the Humber bridge and, beside it and dwarfed by it, the P.S. *Lincoln Castle,* the last coal-fired paddle steamer in the world, now a not-quite-floating restaurant moored on the foreshore at Hessle. Then there are Dunston's shipyard and Hessle Haven, both best visited shoresides and left severely alone by pleasure craft since it is difficult to moor anywhere that seems 'safe' in the usual meaning of that word. There are also the other, almost equally uninspiring, havens of Barrow, Barton and New Holland; the last of these now, after the advent of the new bridge, suddenly old, sad and bereft; seldom visited and little loved.

There are stalwart locals who keep these havens alive, and they have our best wishes, as they have the support of the harbour master of the Humber who looks on it as an important part of his job to ensure that they are neither left to rot nor taken over exclusively by commercial shipping and its heavy require-

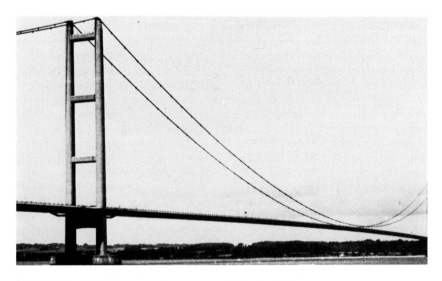

Sooner or later, in this area, you will come across the Humber Bridge . . . or go under it as the case may be.

ments. But until more fortunate times bring nearer hopes of development, they are not places for a casual visit. On a reassuring note, there is also in this area the house of one Paul Berriff, the sea-going television director and cameraman who runs a coastguard station (Humber Bridge CG) from it.

Before the River Hull itself, it is important to point out the presence of that recent institution, Hull Marina. However, before taking the luxury of going ashore, we ought to pay attention to an absolutely remarkable phenomenon of this part of the river: the Hessle Whelps and the Barton Bulldogs. On my first four cruises on the Humber I encountered each of them four times and in progressively aggravating order. They are nasty wavelets in the form of the shortest, sharpest and most vicious whippersnappers that I have experienced in the locality of the east's coastal waters.

Indeed, long before I ever set foot in Kingston-upon-Hull, or, for that matter, set hull into the Humber, I had heard of these strange creatures but did not know for sure what they were. They sound like names for virulent football clubs or roving bands of armed-to-the-teeth footpads. In the event they certainly are virulent and roving, but having nothing at all to do with a game, although there is indeed a tremendous amount of pitching and tossing, as well as slamming, both grand and small and by comparison even the aforementioned footpads seem almost harmless. So what precisely are these bitches of whelps and bulldogs?

Around the River Humber parts of Hessle and Barton there are certain configurations of the river bed that, with the wind in the west and against a flood tide, especially when springs, create such short and sharp broken wave formations that they have been blessed with their unlikely but telling names. They must figure among the most uncomfortable and difficult-to-handle peaks and troughs that any cruising ground can conjure up for the unsuspecting mariner. I can vividly recall one occasion when, inside Hull Marina, the weather was idyllic and even outside it was no more than 3-4 on the Beaufort scale; and that means 'gentle-to-moderate breeze, large wavelets, small waves and fairly frequent horses', conditions that, in most of Britain's rivers and coastal waters, would create no more than a mild disturbance on the surface. This day however carried an especially big spring tide, and the confrontation provided me with one of the most uncomfortable and highly memorable trips of my cruising career. Not only was the wheelhouse constantly aspray, and the hull irregularly but frequently slamming the unconquerable crests, but the waters that swamped over were of such a thick and muddy consistency that they seemed more like cold cocoa than river fluids. And did that stuff find its way around: weeks later, whenever I turned to some partly neglected corner of *Valcon*, I was still being faced with the dried-up remains of that dark brown silt to remind me of those canine furies, the whelps and the bulldogs.

Happily, I can report that there is no such threat inside Kingston-upon-Hull, especially not in its 'new' marina, although there are plenty of good, sound characters who definitely belong to the bulldog breed; and the good, sound capstans that abound in the port certainly still possess their ridges,

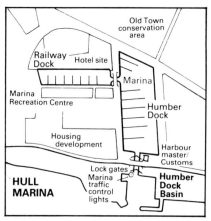

HULL MARINA

Map labels: Old Town conservation area, Railway Dock, Hotel site, Marina, Marina Recreation Centre, Humber Dock, Housing development, Harbour master/Customs, Lock gates, Marina traffic control lights, Humber Dock Basin

KINGSTON-UPON-HULL

Spurn Point 22 miles
Trent Falls 15 miles
Beverley 10 miles
Ferriby 6 miles

Moorings

There are moorings for those with stout hearts, strong craft, stout ropes and strong will inside the River Hull; but the area is extremely busy with extremely rough'n'tough commercial traffic, and although most of the skippers are possessed of hearts of gold, it is a very risky business. For those who are interested, contact Capt. Boylan: ☎ Hull (0482) 22287 or VHF channels 16 and 14, call sign *Drypool Radio*.

Marina

More appealing to the cruising man, especially if waiting a day or two before proceeding up the River Hull, must be the marina: Marina Master Tom Blake: ☎ Hull (0482) 25048 or VHF channel 'M'. The marina is accessible +/− 3 hours HW with 8' maintained inside.

Boatyard

Although there is no actual boatyard within the confines of the marina, because of the nature of Hull itself, you are close to every kind of help that any kind of craft might ever need. If you need anything, contact the marina staff.

Club

Hull Marina Boat Club: Commodore David Towle ☎ Hull (0482) 77978.
Humber Yawl Club, Brough: ☎ Hull (0482) 667224. One of the oldest and friendliest clubs you could happen upon. Visitors are extremely welcome at their establishment, but since their berths always seem to be at bursting point, and they do not have many permanently set aside for visitors, it is only reasonable to ring them well in advance.

Facilities

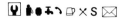

Remarks

The Humber is administered by Capt. Thomas, Harbourmaster of the Humber: Associated British Ports, Kingston House Tower, Bond Street, HU1 3ER. ☎ (0482) 27171. They publish the charts which are essential for anyone cruising these waters.
Vehicle Traffic Service Humber (Call sign *VTS Humber*) work VHF channels 16 and 12 and broadcast local reports at 3 minutes past every odd hour. ☎ Hull (0482) 701787.
Hull itself has all the facilities you could possibly wish for; all it lacks these days is a prosperous fleet of its own fishing vessels.

parallel to the axis, on the drum, to keep the rope, cable or chain from slipping, which, as every schoolboy knows, have always been called whelps.

The city fathers of Kingston are to be congratulated on their marina project. Not only is the place well appointed, and when completed will be one of the foremost marinas in the country, but the officially appointed marina master, one Thomas Blake ('Call me Tom; we don't stand on ceremony very much here,') runs one of the most efficient and friendly establishments I have ever thrown a bowline in. He has a most committed crew, able, friendly and ever

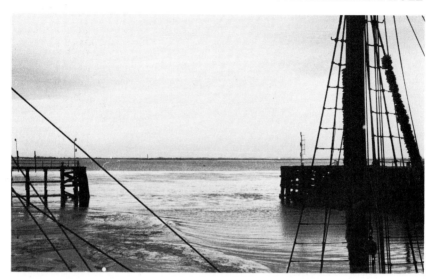

The outer entrance to the marina at Kingston-upon-Hull – and, generally speaking, the River Humber never looks less than bleak . . .

ready, and the spirit of the place is one of happy but not sloppy co-operation. The marina is a place of growth at the time of writing: it is completely in working order and there are excellent facilities there already, but there are targets for expansion well in sight. The tower block amenities (toilets, showers, launderette) are superb, and when the scheme is completed, there will be all the ancillaries that any cruising man might want. There are problems regarding the provision of a lay-by berth in the approach basin (the early attempts came to grief) but it cannot be beyond the wit of Hull men to solve them.

The marina works VHF channel 'M', and I for one have been able to reach them from Keadby, Thorne and Torksey with no mast to provide proper aerial height. Locking is through sector gates that are fail-safe operated and give a really smooth ride, rise and fall, for an operation that can take no more than 130 seconds to gain a level. All craft are logged in and out and asked for ETA's as a standard precaution. Tom's staff can muster French, Dutch, Swedish, Danish, Norwegian and German and have been known to succumb to urgent pleas to 'puppy-sit' poodle offspring. The marina is accessible from ±3 hours HW and a depth of +2.5m O.D.(N) is maintained inside.

Nearby is the hustle and bustle of the wholesale fruit and vegetable dealers although there is no hustling in the pejorative sense; a fresh and frozen fish shop, Smayles, that is a Mecca for fish eaters, be they plain or fancy; the comprehensive delights of the open-air market; and not far away four hostelries of intriguing and varied repute: the Dick Whittington and his Cat, known locally as the Cat, the King William, known locally as the King Billy, the Green Bricks, known locally as the Green Bricks, and the Earl de Grey (known locally).

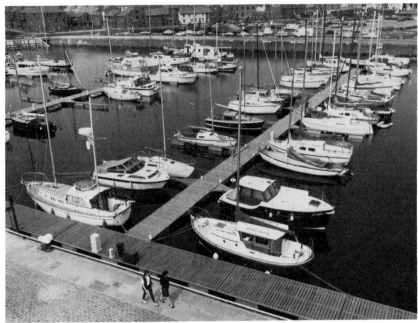

The marina in Kingston-upon-Hull is one of the most up-to-date in the country . . . it is also one of the most welcoming – and, what is more, gets on with the job without fuss or delay.

Captain Thomas who has the unusual-sounding office of harbour master of the Humber was good enough to spend an enormous amount of time and energy ensuring that I got the 'right' picture of the river and his operation and responsibilities. He is a man who is deeply sensible of the needs of the cruising fraternity at large and particularly aware of his obligations to all sensible skippers. He is also, and rightly so, keenly sensitive regarding those who get their kicks from tacking under the bows of big ships or flirting with their sterns; but at the same time he was quick to point out that such behaviour comes only from a minority and is in no way condoned by the local organisations. He reminded me that the Sunk Dredged Channel may not be used without permission from VTS Humber (Vessel Traffic Service Humber: channels 16 and 12) and that in effect pleasure craft are precluded from it. In any case, there are plenty of deep water courses for them, and there is no need for them to be in it at all.

Having worked VTS Humber consistently for help and advice, I was able to compliment him upon their friendly and efficient service. He suggested that, as a general rule, the following should obtain: all pleasure craft for whom the Humber is home water should monitor channel 12 (but not transmit ship to ship as some have done – and indeed as have some professionals who should know better) and visitors should call in and report their presence, position and intentions. VTS Humber broadcasts local reports at 3 minutes past every odd hour; and while listening to their normal working traffic, I was intrigued by their operator's regular use of idiosyncratic phrases: 'All attention' to indicate contact; and 'Well received' to confirm information passed. Nice touches I have not met elsewhere.

Almost immediately next to Hull Marina is the mouth of the River Hull; unmistakably marked by the dominating structure of the concrete towers that support the 200-ton steel gate of the tidal surge barrier. 'Local knowledge' is divided about the attractions of the River Hull for pleasure craft, but there is no doubt that many decry it: because the old port section is packed with rough and tough barges; because the tide can be vicious; because the many bridges can make progress tedious; because there is regular danger of grounding for the stranger; and because there is a tremendous amount of rubbish, especially heavy-duty plastic bags. There is also little doubt that the river is regularly used by the many boats from the Hull Bridge Boat Club and from Beverley Beck, about ten miles from the mouth at the Humber. To get the official low-down from the officiating high-up, I approached the Irish horse's mouth of the harbour master, Captain Patrick Boylan, in his tiny office by Drypool Bridge. He listens on VHF 16 and 14 (call sign: *Drypool radio*) and attends his office in the morning and at tide times. Captain Boylan had no hesitation in recommending his river for the use of pleasure craft. There is a bar at the entrance,

RIVER HULL

Distances
Kingston-upon-Hull (junction with Humber) to Struncheon Hill Lock 20 miles
Tidal throughout
VHF channels 16 and 14 Myton swing bridge, 16 +14 Drypool bridge from 3 hrs before to 1 hr after HW.

Dimensions   *Locks* None
Length unlimited
Beam unlimited
Draught 6'to Grove Hill then decreasing
Air draught –Bridges swing: consult HM

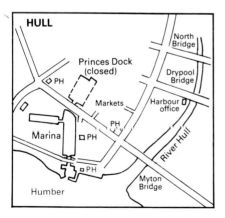

Traffic
There is tremendous commercial traffic within the confines of Hull itself and small craft should only consider staying there in the absence of any other choice. Upstream, the river is used now only by pleasure craft.

Remarks
The tidal river is spanned by ten swing or lift bridges, the hours when these are manned are as follows:

	Hours before HW	Hours after HW
Myton swingbridge		
0600 to 2100 tides	3	1.5
2100 to 0600 tides	2	1
Drypool liftbridge ⎤		
North liftbridge ⎦	3	1.5
Scott Street double leaf liftbridge ⎤		
Sculcoates or Chapman Street liftbridge	2	1
Wilmington high level swingbridge ⎦		
Wilmington high level railway swingbridge ⎤	2	2
Stoneferry swingbridge ⎦		
Sutton Road liftbridge	1.5	3.5

OS Map (1:50,000)
107 Kingston upon Hull

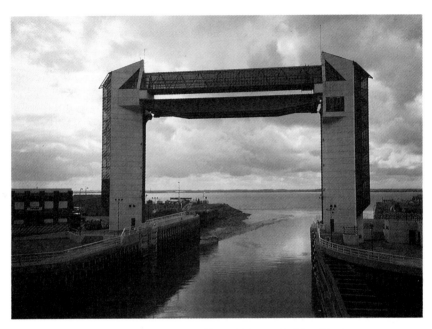

The impressive tidal surge barrier where the River Hull meets the River Humber.

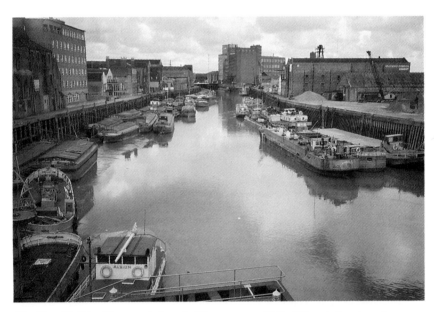

The River Hull is still extremely busy in Kingston-upon-Hull. Although there is no longer any commercial traffic up to Beverley, this part of the river is usually thronged with heavy traffic.

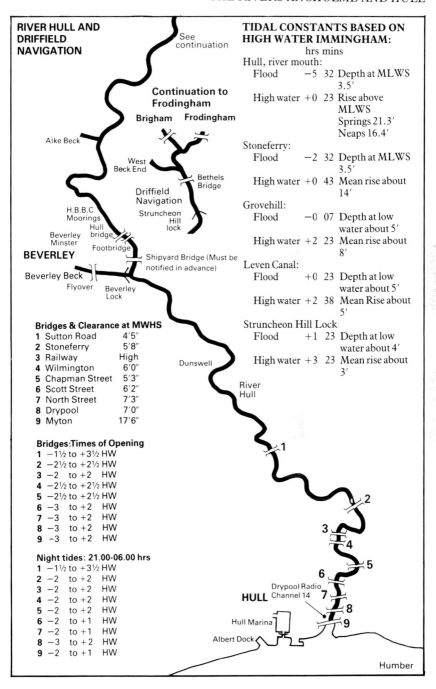

restricting craft to one metre at low water; otherwise the river carries about 1½ metres all the way. The bridges are manned (see data on p.239) and, after prior arrangement with the HM, the signal for opening is 3 blasts. For craft drawing more than one metre, Captain Boylan suggests the river should be entered 2½ hours or so before high water. In the past, there used to be a big barge trade to Beverley, especially toys for Woolworths from Yugoslavia, but now Capt. Boylan speaks of the six wrecks of pleasure craft at Dunswell as more or less symbolic of a trade that seems never likely to return.

The lower stretches of the River Hull are not for pleasure cruising. The rate of knots and the rate of traffic, combined with the number and height of the bridges all make manoeuvring just that bit too difficult for mere pleasure. Most people use the river because they want to get somewhere – and that means the upper reaches for Beverley and Driffield. However, before we leave Hull itself, there is more to be said about the place for it has a deep and dyed-in-the-wool history.

The ancient port has over the centuries been granted over 30 charters and letters patent, the first of which emanated from Edward I in 1299 – and he is the king whose 'Kyngs-town' it first became. Of special interest to cruising folk will be the Maritime Heritage Weekends that the city promotes. I have tried them and found them to be of great interest, especially if you are looking for a couple of days of something different to entertain mutinous crew members. This is what Hull says about them:

'The story of Hull's maritime past runs like a thread through the mercantile history of England. For at least 800 years, generation after generation of Hull men and women have won a living from the sea and by trading with the world.

Hull was the country's third port as long ago as the 14th century and Hull 'shipmen' are even mentioned by Chaucer. Hull ships were sent to support Drake against the Spanish Armada, and were troop carriers on numerous other military expeditions. Hull whalers roamed the Arctic and their successors made the port England's deep-sea fishing capital. In the 19th century the quality of its shipyards persuaded the Czar to have not one but two steam yachts built in Hull.

In this historic setting a new heritage weekend has been prepared that will appeal to all those with a love for the sea and our island history. For any weekend there is a Martitime Heritage Bargain Break in Hull at £50; and this includes two nights, at the award-winning Waterfront Hotel and all VAT and service charges.'

Kingston-upon-Hull has long been regarded as one of our great sea ports. Over the centuries it has traded with the world: from wool, corn and wines in mediaeval times, to, more recently, vehicles, machinery, building materials and basic commodities. As long ago as the 16th century it was known for its whaling expertise and, during the 20th century, became famous as a deep-sea fishing centre.

Although Hull has been a port for almost as long as people have lived on the site, the first Royal recognition of its importance came in 1382 when King Richard II granted it port status. Among the many Royal charters that have been given to the city, was one granted by Henry VI in 1447. This allowed the Corporation the right to elect 'a suitable and discreet man, according to the wise discretion of the Aldermen' to be Admiral of the Humber. And while it has never been laid down specifically that the person elected is to be the Lord Mayor, nevertheless, that person has always by custom been so appointed.

Within the area under his jurisdiction (the whole of the Humber) his authority was above that of all the other Admirals of England. He was to receive 'all the profits of office' including the rights of wreck, flotsam and jetsam, salvage, royal fish such as whales, sturgeon and porpoises, and goods taken from pirates and enemy ships. There was also the Admiral's court, which he held to try all offences relating to ships and shipping matters.

The principal features of the maritime trail itself are the Maritime Museum which possesses galleries on whaling, scrimshaw (the art of carving in whalebone), fishing, shipping and inland waterways; the Hull Marina; Wilberforce House, which commemorates the fight against the slave trade by its namesake who was born in Hull; and a variety of merchants' houses, warehouses and riverside quays. There is also dinner aboard the *Lincoln Castle*, the last coal-fired paddle steamer to operate as a ferry. She now lies in a specially constructed berth in the shadow of the great Humber bridge, not far away from the foreshore site where the Ferriby Plank Boats were discovered, dating navigation on the Humber back to the Bronze Age.

There is a heritage tour of the surrounding countryside with a maritime flavour: Beverley, once a port of greater importance than Hull; Hornsea, with its Mere; Bridlington; and then on to Flamborough Head. The octagonal chalk lighthouse, standing about 1000 yards inland, was built in 1674 by Sir John Clayton, and in those days was lit by a fire in the cresset in the tower. The present-day brick lighthouse was built in 1806, and its light (Fl(4)15s65m29M Horn(2)90s) is 3½ million candle power. The fog signal station was built in 1859 and a cannon was fired in fog until 1877 when a rocket was used. The nearby toposcope was erected to commemorate the 180th anniversary of the battle with the ´now lightly fantastic and totally notorious´ John 'Paul' Jones. On the top there are some incongruous records of distances from various parts of the world to Flamborough Head. A few cobles still use North Landing; but in the past there used to be many, with the fishermen often keeping a boat at each landing (north and south) so they could get to sea no matter where the wind came from. The old lifeboat station was built at South Landing in 1871 and closed in 1938. It is now used as a coble boathouse. The first ever lifeboat was *The St. Michael's, Paddington*. It was here that it was intended in 1975 to build a marina for about 500 boats; but the plans never got off the ground. The days of merchant adventurers may be long gone in the city of Kingston-upon-Hull, but there are still plenty of adventurous merchants, in all kinds of office, from freelance entrepreneurs to the Admiral of the Humber and his admirable officers and crew.

DRIFFIELD CANAL

Moorings
Bethell's Bridge Boat Club moorings are to be found above the swing bridge. Mooring space for visitors can usually be found. ☎ Hull (0482) 442884. There are also some visitors' moorings to be found at Frodingham Landing. The two clubs are the Driffield Navigation Amenities Association and the Bethell's Bridge one.

Boatyard
Beverley Beck is a small canal locked off the River Hull. It has been used for many years until recently by commercial barges plying to and from Beverley. It is the home of the Humber Keel *Comrade* which is owned by the Humber Keel and Sloop Preservation Society. There are boatyards in business in the Beck, repairing small and medium craft.

Remarks
Do not take liberties by assuming that you are entitled to moor; there is no general right of mooring. Always ask permission.
Watch your choice of moorings. Avoid mooring close to Hemphole water supply intake or adjacent to the nature reserves on West Beck and at Pulfin Bog. Moor securely: the water level or flow may fluctuate; allow for this when mooring up.
Traffic in the River Hull is very busy during the week and Saturday mornings; but there can still be barges and coasters moving during the rest of the weekend. The flow in the River Hull can exceed 6 knots at times especially on the last of the spring ebb. Always keep to the centre of the river, especially at bridges and from Stoneferry Bridge to the sewerage outfall as there are submerged piles on both banks in places. After the next bend and under the electricity pylon at Dunswell there are several sunken craft in centre and on port side. Keeping to starboard after makes the journey to Beverley straightforward. There are cranes and old barges to port as Beverley Beck comes into sight. Craft may lay on the concrete wharf to wait for the lock.

STRUNCHEON HILL LOCK

Registration for craft using the canal:
Driffield Navigation Ltd,
70 Middle St South,
Driffield YO2S 7QF

Restricting dimensions 58' x 14'6"
Rise and fall Maximum 8' on a low tide
Hand operated • BWB pattern lock key required.
Boater operated •
Windlass required • BWB square drive for bottom lock; keys for top lock at gate
Facilities nearby
⚓
🖂 S ♪
3 miles and 10 minutes walk

Remarks
No other locks are as yet operable on the Driffield Navigation. The waterway is navigable up to Brigham and North Frodingham, where up to 40' craft can turn. There is a swing bridge at Hempholme, just under a mile above the lock. The best time to go up the River Hull for this canal is about 3 hours before HW with draught up to 3' (three feet). Deeper draught boats should allow a further ½ hour at least. It is prudent to ease off for all the bridges just in case you are not sure of the clearance, as the current flows pretty quickly. Going downstream, for the safest journey through Hull, leave Beverley about 4¼ hours before HW arriving Sutton road bridge about 3 hours before HW. This allows you to push the tide and so retain full control through the bridge. Always keep your eyes open for commercial craft and overtake only when signalled to do so.
Local information may be obtained by phoning the following:
Mr. P. Kissagizlis ☎ Hull (0482) 444588
Mr. A. Ball ☎ Hull (0482) 442884
Mr. D. Madin ☎ Hull (0482) 846083

However, no matter how magnetically appealing or hypnotically fascinating Hull and its features and folk may be, in the end, our concern here is to consider the navigation of the River Hull and find out where it will take us. I have already mentioned the bridges and the control office of the harbour master of the River Hull at Drypool, by the bridge; and Captain Boylan is the man for any visitor to contact well before making an initial visit. There are also others possessed of that invaluable commodity 'local knowledge' and prepared to share it with visitors wanting to make their way through the city parts of the river and on up to Beverley and/or Driffield. They are: Alan Ball, 12 Weighton Grove, Hull (Tel: Hull (0482) 442884), who not only has local knowledge, but also has local contacts through the Driffield Navigation Amenities Association and the commissioners of the navigation. Roger Hargreaves, 14-16 King Street, Cottingham, N. Humberside, (Tel: Hull (0482) 849580),who runs a navigation and seamanship school from his own craft but who will also co-operate with visitors in putting them or keeping them 'right', works his own boats from Albert Dock, Hull, and from Grimsby Fish Dock.

Once out of the conurbation that is Hull (although that will take a little time to achieve, for it stretches towards the north more than somewhat) the scenery changes dramatically and shows some of the best countryside that east Yorkshire has to offer: scattered farms, small brick-built villages, attractive market towns, windmills and church towers, solid and square against the winter gales, are all actual and symbolic landmarks in this wide open land of even wider horizons.

Beverley and Driffield must be the main objectives of any visitor coming up the River Hull. The approaches to both are locked: the first at Beverley Beck, leaving no more than ¾ mile to get into the town; and the second at Struncheon Hill Lock after which there are eleven miles to Great Driffield. The Driffield Navigation runs from its eponymous home town to a junction with the River Hull at Aike; and running off it there is also Frodingham Beck, with a distance of about a mile, and West Beck with a navigably doubtful couple of miles. There is also an intriguing section in a kind of no man's land, currently nominated a free navigation, that runs from Sculcoates Goate to Aike; after this stretch the River Hull is deemed to be part and parcel of the port of Hull.

Any visitor drawing more than a metre should make contact with one of the two gentlemen mentioned above, indeed, it is a good idea for any and every visitor to do so in the first place. Alan Ball will also be able to provide you with a copy of *A Guide to the Driffield Navigation* which goes into all the details of the past and present of the navigation, and is required reading for any skipper making his first pass through these parts. Once upstream, the joys of the waterways are tremendous; but there is no doubt that the approach through the city reaches of the River Hull needs well-found craft with well-motivated skippers and well-informed crews plus as many well-wishers as can be mustered.

For those with a mind to plan ahead, here are the relevant details:

LOCK DIMENSIONS

Grovehill	65' x 17.5' x 6'
Struncheon Hill	60' x 14' x 4'

INDEX

Acaster Malbis, 200
Acaster Selby, 198
Aire & Calder Navigation,
    141-176
    authorities, 143
    details, 141, 142-3
    distances, table of, 144
    plan, 142
Aire, River, 152, 156
Aldwarke Lock, 132, 134
Ancholme, River, 231-4
    authorities, 221
    distances, table of, 225
Anchor Pit Flood Lock, 171
Anton's Gowt, 32-4
    Lock, 33
Apex lighthouse, 67, 68,
    177, 219
authorities, 5-7

Bain, Old River, 38
Bank Dole Lock, 174, 175
Bardney, 42-4
    Lock, 43-4
Barlby Reach, 197
Barmby Lock, 214, 216
Barmby Tidal Barrage, 213,
    214
Barnby Dun, 123
    Lift Bridge, 123, 124
Barton, 235
Battye Cut Lock, 169
Battye Flood Lock, 169
Bawtry, 99
Beal Lock, 175, 176
Beningborough, 208
Beverley, 245
Birkwood Lock, 162
Bishopthorpe, 202
Blacktoft Jetty, 66, 67, 145,
    181-2, 185
books, recommended, 16
Boothferry Bridge, 191
Boroughbridge, 210
Boston, 23-32
    details, 28
    Lock, 28
Bramwith, 117
    Lock, 117
    Swing Bridge, 117

Brandy Wharf, 233-4
Branston Island, 44
Brayford Pool, 49-52
Brigg, 233
Brighouse Locks, 171
British Waterways Board, iv,
    7
    Code of Conduct, 9-13
    water points, 14-15
Broad Cut, 166
    Low and Top Locks, 167
Broadreach Flood Lock, 163
Brookfoot Lock, 171
Broomfleet Island, 223
Brough Haven, 224, 226
Bulholme Lock, 155
Burton-upon-Stather, 71

Calder & Hebble, 142-3,
    163, 164-73
    details, 165-6
    distances, table of, 165
    plan, 166
Castle Mills Lock, 203
Castleford Junction Lock,
    155, 161
Castleford, 154-6
Cawood, 197-8
Chapel Hill, 34-7
charts, recommended, 17
Cherry Willingham, 45
Chesterfield Canal, 98-9,
    101-2
    distances, table, of, 98
Clayworth, 101
Clifton Bridge, 203
Clifton Ings, 206
Colwick Park, 93
commercial wharves, 17-21
conversion tables, 21-2
Cooper Bridge Flood Lock,
    170
Cooper Bridge Lock, 170
Cottingwith Lock, East
    (Swing Bridges), 217
Cowbridge Lock, 59
Cromwell Bottom, 170
    Lock, 171
Cromwell, 86-7
    Lock, 87

Derwent, River, 213-17
Dewsbury Arm, 168
distances, table of,
    main routes, 4
Dogdyke, 34-8
Don Aqueduct, 121
Doncaster, 126-7
    Lock, 127
Don, River, 123-4, 141, 143
Double Bridges, 131, 135
Double Locks, 168
Drakeholes Tunnel, 101
Driffield Navigation, 241,
    244-5
Drinsey Nook, 54
Drypool, 239
Dunston Hill Swing Bridge,
    117
Dutch River, 124, 141, 143

Eastwood, lock, 132, 134
Elland Lock, 172
Elvington (Sutton) Lock,
    216

Fall Ings Lock, Wakefield,
    161, 163
Farndon, 90-1
Ferriby Sluice, 229, 230-32
Ferriby, North, 228
Ferriby, South, 228,
    229-32
    Lock, 231, 232
Ferrybridge, 152-4
    Lock, 154
Figure of Three Locks,
    166-8
Fishlake, 117
Fishpond Lock, 159
Fiskerton (Trent), 91
Fiskerton (Witham), 45
Five Mile Bridge, 45
Fossdyke Navigation, 33,
    55-8
Foss, River, 203, 207
Frank Price Lock
    (Eastwood), 132, 134
Frodingham Beck, 245

Gainsborough, 82-3
Ganny Lock, 171
Gardham Lock (Swing
   Bridges), 217
Glory Hole (High Bridge),
   47-9
Godknow Swing Bridge,
   108, 109
Goole, 141, 143-7, 183-9
   details, 186
   docking signals, 187
   Docks, 186-7
   pilots, 185, 189
   radio information, 185
Grand Sluice, 29-30
Greenwood Flood Lock, 169
Greenwood Lock, 168
Gringley-on-the-Hill, 101
Gunthorpe, 92-3
   Lock, 92

Haddlesey Lock, West, 176
Haddlesey, West, Chapel,
   East, 175
Halifax Arm, 170
Hazelford Lock, 91-2
Heck, 148-51
Hessle Haven, 234, 235
Hexthorpe, 127
Holme Locks, 93, 94
Holmes Lock, 136
Horbury, 166
Horncastle, 34
   Canal, 34-5, 38-9
Howden Dyke Island, 191
Huddersfield Broad Canal,
   143
Hull, River, 239-45
   authorities, 221
   details, 239
   distances, table of, 225
   plan, 241
   tidal constants, 241
Hull, see Kingston-Upon-
   Hull
Humber Anchorage, 66
Humber, River, 219-22,
   224-31, 234-9, 243
   Bridge, 234
   pilots, 185
   plans, 221, 226-7
   radio information, 185,
      238-9

Ickles Lock, 134
Idle, River, 78, 97-101
   distances, table of, 98

Jordan Lock, 136

Keadby Canal, Stainforth
   and, 103-117
Keadby, 71-2, 103, 106-8
   details, 76, 106
   Lock, 73-7, 103, 106-7
   key to symbols, 7
Kilnhurst Lock, 132, 133
King George Bridge,
   Keadby, 72
Kings Road Lock, 162
Kingston-Upon-Hull,
   235-40, 242-3
   details, 236
Kippax Lock, 157
Kirk Lane Bridge, 120
Kirkhouse Green Bridge,
   120
Kirklees Low Lock, 171
Kirklees Top Lock, 171
Kirkstead Bridge, 39-40
Knaith, 83
Knostrop Fall Lock, 159
Knottingley, 151-2
Kyme Eau, 34-7

Langrick, 34
Langthorpe, 210
Ledgard Bridge Flood Lock,
   169
Leeds, 123, 160-1
   City Lock, 160
Lemonroyd Lock, 157
Lendal Bridge, 203
licences, pleasure boat, 16
Lincoln, 46-51
Linton, 208, 209, 210
locks
   number of, 4
   use of, 11-13
Long Lee Lock, 172
Long Sandall Lock, 123
Low Lane Bridge, 119

maps, recommended, 17
Market Weighton Canal,
   220, 222-4
Martin Dales, 39
Maud's Swing Bridge, 109,
   111

Meadow Lane Lock, 93-4,
   95-6
Medge Hall Swing Bridge,
   108,109
Mexborough, 131
   Low Lock, 131, 133
   Top lock, 131, 133
Milby Lock, 211
Millbank Lock, 168
Misson, 99
Misterton, 101
Moor's Swing Bridge, 109,
   111
Morse Lock, 102
Myton, 212

Naburn, 199-202
   Locks, 199-201
Nether Poppleton, 206
New Junction Canal,
   118-122
Newark, 88-90
   Lock, Nether and Town,
      90
Nidd, River, 208
North Muskham, 87
Northeast Waterways,
   system map, 2
Nottingham, 4, 93-7
Nun Monkton, 208-10

Ocean Lock, 146, 183-4, 187
Ordnance Survey maps, 17
Ouse Bridge, 203
Ouse Bridge, 191
Ouse, Yorkshire, 177-212
   authorities, 179
   details, 179-80
   distances, table of, 180
   navigation marks, 187
   plan, 178
   radio information, 185
Oxclose Lock, 210, 211

Park Nook Lock, 172
Pocklington Canal, 213
Pollington Lock, 148, 149
pump out locations, 14

Ramsden's Swing Bridge,
   162
Read's Island, 226
Red Doles Lock, 173
registration certificates, 16
Retford, 101-2

Ripon, 210
Ripon Canal, 212
Rotherham, 126, 132-3
 Lock, 134

Salterhebble,
 Locks, Nos. 1-9, 172-3
Saltmarshe, 182
sanitary stations, 14
Saxilby, 53-4
Scarborough Bridge, 203
Selby Canal, 142-3, 174-6,
 196
 plan, 174
Selby, 143, 175, 176,
 194-7
 Bridges, 193-4, 195,
 196,197
 Lock, 175, 176, 192-3
Sheffield & South Yorkshire
 Navigation, 103 –139
 authorities, 105
 details, 104-5
 distances, table of, 105
 plans, 104, 125
Sheffield, 138-9
 Canal Basin, 123, 136,
 138-9
 Canal, 122-139
Shepley Bridge Lock, 170
Shortferry, 43-4
Skeldergate Bridge, 203
Skelton Railway Bridge, 206
Sleaford, 34
Southfield Reservoir, 122
Southrey, 41
Sowerby Bridge, 170
Sprotbrough, 128-9, 131
 Lock, 128-9
Stainforth, 117
Stamp End Lock, 46-7
Stanley Ferry, 162
Stockwith, West, 78-82, 97
 Lock, 79-80, 99
Stoke Bardolph, 93
Stoke Lock, 93, 94
Strawberry Island, 126
Struncheon Hill Lock, 244
Sutton Lock, 213, 215- 6
Swale Nab, 210
Swale, River, 212
Swinton, 132
Sykehouse Lock, 120
Sykehouse Road Bridge, 120

Tattershall, 34-5, 38-9
 Bridge, 38
Thorne, 109-116
 details, 111
 Lock, 111
Thornes Flood Lock, 167
Thornes Locks, 167
Thornhill Flood Lock, 168
tidal differences, 8
Tinsley Flight, 136-8
Top Lane Bridge, 119
Torksey, 54-8, 84-6
 Lock, 55, 56-7, 86
Trent Anchorage, 66
Trent Falls, 69, 178
Trent, River, 61-97
 authorities, 63
 BWB navigation notes,
 64-5
 details, 64
 distances, table of, 63
 eagre, 70
 plan, 62
 VHF radio channels, 69

Ure, River, 210-12

Vazon Swing Bridge, 108
VHF radio at locks, 15

Waddington (Swinton)
 Lock, 132, 133
Wakefield Arm, 161
Wakefield, 163-4
 Flood Lock, 167
Washingborough, 45
water points, BWB, 14-15
Weighton (Humber) Lock,
 222
West Beck, 245
Westwick Lock, 211
Wharfe,River, 198
wharves, freight, 17-21
Whitley, 148, 151
 Lock, 151, 152
Whitsunday Pie Lock, 102
Whitton, 224
Wikewell Bridge, 111
Winteringham Haven, 224,
 226
Wiseton, 101
Witham & Fossdyke, 23-60
 authorities, 24
 details, 25
 dimensions, 25

distances, table of, 25
plan, 24
Witham Navigable Drains,
 32-3, 58-60
Witham, River, 23-55
 plan, Boston to Lincoln,
 26
Woodhall Spa, 39-41
Woodlesford, 156-9
 Lock, 157
Woodnook Lock, 162
Woodside Mills Lock, 172
Worksop, 102

Yorkshire Canal, South,
 124-5
 *see also Sheffield & South
 Yorkshire Navigation*
York, 203-6, 207